In memory of
Cathy
(1963 - 2017)
May her valiant struggle not have been in vain,
so that her story will help other cancer patients
to get effective treatment and be cured of the disease.

LIFELINE

The Case for Effective Cancer Immunotherapy

T.S.Aguilar

LIFELINE – The Case for Effective Cancer Immunotherapy
A T.S.Aguilar book
First edition: 2020

ISBN: 978-0-9687711-3-6

Preamble

First of all I advise every reader that this book should not be construed as medical advice - repeat - it is not medical advice for cancer treatment. It does not propagate a miraculous cure or suggest consulting soothsayers who claim to have cured thousands of terminally ill cancer patients. It presents an incisive look at current cancer treatment, what is wrong with it, why orphan medications that could improve the outcome of conventional treatment are denied clinical trials, and the ongoing research and development of immunotherapies that provide a ray of hope for a cancer cure in the near future.

Now you may well ask what moves a guy without medical training to write about cancer, one of the most complex diseases to befall humanity. It started as a therapy of writing down my wife Cathy's case history of struggling with the disease and my concurrent search for a cure. Nineteen-month after she was diagnosed my wife succumbed to cancer when we were denied the medicine that could have prolonged her life and in the best case cured her. It is a story that is probably familiar to most families and caregivers who have lost a loved one to the disease and is equally familiar to the millions of patients searching and hoping for a cure.

I continued researching current cancer treatment, and it became apparent that the prescribed and administered therapies and medications fail to have any curative effect for millions of cancer patients. Hence and not just by chance, Big Pharma's medicine that results in the death of over nine million cancer patients globally a year after an allegedly "effective" treatment came into focus. There is practically no cure for cancer at present because the eight and a half million "survivors" have on average about five years of progression free survival before the cancer recurs in a more aggressive form and ends with the death of the patients.

My research also shed some light on malpractice and corruptibility of institutes and practitioners as well as the media's promotion of alleged advances in conventional cancer treatment.

The negative and depressing outcome of the research of current cancer treatment moved me to search for new and unconventional treatments and medications and concluded with an investigation of curative therapies that provide hope for all people afflicted with cancer, directly and indirectly. The outcome was the case for effective immunotherapy to heal patients of their cancer.

It resulted in a positive outlook that should give hope to all people diagnosed with cancer to be cured of the disease for good in the foreseeable future. It is still some way to go and the scientists and researchers will want to learn much more about cancer and the immune system before a great and ultimate medical breakthrough will be achieved. The good news is that there is indeed light at the end of the tunnel and by all accounts it is not an oncoming train.

The critical wording describing dithering medics and useless therapies may look like a condemnation of the health care systems of the two countries where my wife was diagnosed and ultimately failed to be treated effectively. But it is not! The health care systems of most other countries are not any better and in many cases far worse. It doesn't matter if a health care system is public or private, universal or based on individual health insurance policies. All of them are inadequate to provide effective curative cancer treatment and prevent the death of millions of patients.

Several hurdles will have to be taken to improve health care. Among them are better work conditions and salaries of health care workers to attract more young people into these professions and alleviate present day shortages. The financing of immunotherapy research and development has to be increased. The bureaucracy that hinders the acceptance of

2

researchers' trial results as relevant needs to be overcome as well as Big Pharma's lack of interest in and its active hindrance of finding and implementing a cancer cure. The epidemics and pandemics of the recent past have confirmed the inadequacies of current health care policies. It begs the question if any country needs more bureaucrats to administer its health care system than medical practitioners and yet at salaries that would make nurses swoon with happiness if they received the bureaucrats' remuneration in recognition of their work.

Politicians of all stripes should agree to raise the health care budgets instead of slashing them and provide a functioning, comprehensive universal health care. It should include dental, ocular, and auditory treatments needed mainly by old people who are also the age group most vulnerable to cancer. It has to be recognised that only a population whose health care is assured without driving it into bankruptcy and poverty can achieve the happiness it deserves and be fully productive.

Governments should restrain their bureaucracy, promote and support medical research and development at universities, and stop whining about how much health care costs. Instead they should consider it an investment into social cohesion that is lost due to the lack of effective care for the sick and elderly.

In short, the book is a summary of my multi-year investigation of medical practice, the health care industry, and Big Pharma. It is a critical assessment of conventional cancer treatments based on my experience as caregiver of both my mother and my wife who were diagnosed with and succumbed to cancer. It concludes with insights into the research of techniques and therapies that enhance immunotherapy, the manipulation and strengthening of the human immune system, and its facilitation to eradicate cancer cells without side effects.

Thus, writing this essay was like passing through a dark valley of death into the glimmer of hope of a new day.

Cathy's Case History

This is the case history of the conventional cancer treatment that failed my wife and led ultimately to what I regard as her untimely death.

In early May 2016, my wife was diagnosed with cancer. We resided and worked in Saudi Arabia at the time. The nineteen months that followed until her death in Canada in early December 2017 was a roller coaster of emotions.

Brief euphoric moments of hope were shattered one after another. The surgery two specialists had recommended when they were consulted for a second opinion was declared out of the question by the windbag of a doctor who was in charge of her treatment and had misdiagnosed her cancer. The anticancer treatments with chemo- and radiotherapy did not have any positive effect, and in the end the doctors refused to prescribe the medication that might have saved or at least prolonged Cathy's life. Instead she was pumped full of Fentanyl, the opioid of infamy in the opioid crisis of North America and other parts of the world.

The loss of a loved one to cancer is always a tragedy. When my wife and partner of 25 years died, overwhelming grief took hold, especially because Cathy had been only a step away from potential relief if not a cure. Thus, my grief was laced with bitterness and anger.

Doubts continue to gnaw away at me to this day, doubts if I had done enough to help save her life, and if I couldn't have been more forceful to demand the treatment that would have eased her suffering, extended her life expectancy, and potentially cured her of the cancer.

However, obtaining the medication for various types of cancer that serves at least as an adjunct in the apoptosis of cancer cells is going to be difficult in most countries. The health care authorities simply shut their eyes to the research done around the globe and will not permit the prescription of a drug that has not yet undergone a clinical trial on their home turf despite the documented scientific proof of its efficacy achieved in other countries.

The doctors that were licensed to prescribe the well-known and very affordable adjunct medication we wanted, ignored or rejected the scientific evidence about its curative effect, and refused to consider it even as an analgesic, although in that capacity it is prescribed and administered.

During the entire episode of the misdiagnosis, delays, and failed treatments I made mistakes because I was totally unprepared. Neither Cathy nor I had ever thought of suffering cancer, prepared for it, or considered what needed to be done in case it happened. Also, we had faith in most of the doctors we consulted and trusted them, which in retrospect turns out to have been a bad mistake because we couldn't tell the trustworthy medical practitioners apart from the blowhards who should have their license withdrawn and be banished from working in the field of health care.

In the hope that Cathy's case history will help you to avoid our mistakes and be treated more successfully, I accentuate our mistakes and failures for you to pursue a course of action that could result in a more fortunate outcome.

Among the medics we consulted stand out the doctors and especially the nurse practitioners that truly cared. I express my deeply felt gratitude to them. They did everything in their power to help but were prevented by the bureaucracy of the current health care systems to get the treatment or prescribe and administer the medication that was necessary. They are proof that competent and dedicated medical professionals do exist and can be trusted. Unfortunately, most of them can be and are overruled by domineering colleagues who quite evidently care more about polishing their egos and very little about the positive outcome of saving a life.

These overbearing medics we had the bad fortune to consult disappear in a nebula of full-throated claims and helplessly flailing arms as well as their conceited, jingoistic dismissals of research done and curative results achieved in what are to them foreign countries and therefore irrelevant.

Those flailing medics are reminiscent of Johann Andreas Eisenbart, a doctor of the 18th century. Decades after his death, medical students wrote the following satirical poem about his controversial treatments:

> *I am Doctor Eisenbart,*
> *treat people with my healing art.*
> *I can make the blind to walk,*
> *and the lame again to talk!*
> *The sexton's son at Dideldum*
> *I gave ten pounds of opium.*
> *He fell asleep, years passed away,*
> *and still he sleeps until this day.*

The last three lines of the poem are reminiscent of the treatment my wife received in the end. Reading them, I can only wonder if all that much has changed in the 'Health Care Industry' since the 18th century.

How will today's health care and medical practices be seen in a couple of centuries or so - if humanity should survive for that long? Will there again be some medical students writing satirical poems about stupidly obstinate and ignorant medics of today? Will future generations have reason to laugh about today's medical practices? One can only hope for the sake of humanity that it will be the case.

But let's start at the beginning.

Suddenly and Unexpected...

It was bright and sunny morning in Riyadh, Saudi Arabia, on Wednesday, 4th May 2016. My wife Cathy and I had got up early and we were ready for our respective work. Cathy taught at a medical college and I worked on the design of a geothermal power system.

Cathy was in a happy mood. The final exam papers she had prepared for intermediate level female students had not only been accepted the previous day but were also commended for their cultural sensitivity. She looked as radiant as ever and nobody could have expected what would unfold in the course of the day.

We lived with our cat Sparky in a single-family villa in a housing compound, a closed and guarded community complex by the name of Al Yamama ('The Dove'). It is located approximately 15 km (10 miles) from the campus of the King Saud University for Health Sciences, Cathy's place of work.

The university is part of a huge medical complex, King Abdullah Medical City. It is not an independent city, but a complex in the east of Riyadh with hospitals, housing for medical staff, shops, restaurants, banks, and the colleges of the university. It is run and financed by the National Guard of Saudi Arabia. The medical facilities are freely accessible and free of charge to anyone with National Guard health insurance - and Saudi royalty, of course.

When we were ready to go to work, I drove her as I did every workday in our sub-compact rental car through the hectic morning traffic while cautiously avoiding drivers who appeared to be on a suicide mission.

Believe me, driving in Saudi Arabia and especially in Riyadh was not a lot of fun. Some people compared it to a bumper car rally where traffic signs and speed limits are ignored, and traffic lights serve to illuminate intersections. Cathy had often wondered why any woman would want to drive a car in that city, that country. Well, now the Saudi women can drive and hopefully they contribute to a more sedate driving style and some consideration for the other traffic participants.

I dropped her off at the gates of the Women's Medical College that no man, except technical maintenance staff under guard, is permitted to enter. I wished her a pleasant day and promised to pick her up after classes.

I returned home where I worked on the final touches of my project that I was to present to some rich knobs for the financing of the prototype.

Absorbed in my work I didn't notice a taxi pulling up in front of our villa about midday. I was surprised to see Cathy come into the house and noticed the distinct yellow discolouration of her face.

Wanting to know what had happened to her, she told me that her superior had noticed the rapid change of her complexion and sent her home on suspicion that she had a sudden case of jaundice as a result of the lunch she had eaten in the cafeteria.

Not familiar with the cause of jaundice, I had no idea how that could have happened so suddenly or how one sandwich could be the cause. We decided to go immediately to the hospital to have her medical condition diagnosed.

The First Misdiagnosis

I dropped Cathy off at the regular medical ward, not the emergency ward when she assured me that she was still feeling fine.

I waited in the lobby for her return. It is depressing to sit in a public waiting area where hundreds of people with all sorts of ailments hobble past. And it got worse when Cathy returned. She looked distraught when she conveyed the doctor's diagnosis.

He had dismissed her with his conclusion that the jaundice was caused by the excessive consumption of alcohol. He had stated to know what he was talking about from his years of study in Glasgow and Liverpool, the alleged binge drinking capitals of Scotland and England!

He insisted that Cathy's problem was the onset of cirrhosis of the liver that would go away as soon as she stopped boozing. That was his experience with all the other expatriates he treated every day. Or so he claimed.

That sot hadn't even listened to Cathy's argument that we had never in our life been binge drinking and she hadn't consumed any alcohol in more than twelve years. He insisted that all expatriates are alcoholics and that was that.

When Cathy pointed him out to me as he waltzed through the lobby, I got the picture. He was not dressed like a Saudi and thus it was fair to assume that he was an expatriate from some Middle Eastern country. His puffy face, bulbous red nose, and droopy eyelids provided the appearance of an alcoholic on his way home for some serious drinking to get blotto on home-distilled hooch.

Challenging that pompous so-called doctor in the public waiting area would have been counterproductive. Instead we arranged an appointment for the next day and insisted that it had to be a Saudi doctor, not another expatriate.

10

A Meticulous Exam

After that disastrous first consultation, we hoped that the next doctor would not project his own addictions onto others and know that quite a few people don't like to pickle their brains.

As arranged, the appointment was with a Saudi doctor, not an expatriate. Cathy underwent a lengthy interview and a thorough exam on Thursday, 5th May 2016.

Methodically the doctor excluded various origins of the jaundice: no alcohol, no careless consumption of dubious food and drink, and no swimming in parasitic flatworm infested fresh water. That appeared to exclude cirrhosis and hepatitis, which still had to be ascertained, but it was most definitely not bilharzia, which can cause jaundice and is sometimes mistaken for liver cancer. Bilharzia - also known as snail fever - is caused by parasitic flatworms called schistosomes. It causes liver damage, kidney failure, infertility, and bladder cancer.

He ordered a blood test and scheduled a computer tomography scan (CT scan) for Monday, 9th May 2016, to get a clear picture of what the problem was with her liver.

The hepatitis and cirrhosis tests turned out to be negative, i.e. the diseases were not detected. But the scan showed two large tumours, one below the liver, and one on the spleen. The doctor ordered a biopsy of the tumour below the liver but not for the growth on the spleen, which he presumed to be benign on account of its shape and colour. Several months later it turned out to have been a correct assumption. A biopsy of the growth on the spleen done in Canada provided proof that it was benign.

The biopsy of the tumour underneath the liver was done on Thursday, 12th May 2016, and Cathy was given a diagnosis appointment for Thursday, 19th May 2016.

Devastating News

On the day of her diagnosis appointment I brought Cathy into the good care of the doctor and proceeded on my usual tour of shops and supermarkets in preparation for the weekend. I felt confident that this doctor was on the ball and would assess her illness correctly. Unfortunately, he was "only" a general practitioner and the two consultations with him should remain all she ever saw of this competent and dedicated professional.

Shortly before midday I arrived at a shopping mall when Cathy called me. She was crying and told me the doctor's diagnosis. He had consulted with cancer specialists who claimed that it was hepatocellular carcinoma. I didn't understand what that meant until she used the layman's term: Liver Cancer.

Well, she might as well have hit me in the head with a rubber mallet - it would have had the same effect as this devastating news.

All I could mutter at that moment was for her to stay calm. I rambled on about the advances of cancer research and recited some vague news I had read some time ago without having paid too much attention to the details or wording of the report that some pharma company claimed to have developed the panacea that humanity had been waiting for to finally beat cancer.

I cut the shopping spree short, drove home as fast as possible, and started a search of the Internet for liver cancer treatments and to help me understand Cathy's illness.

I had to learn everything and anything there is to know about the liver and its function. It was crucial to find out more than I knew about the location of this vital organ and that one cannot live without it.

Gaining an Insight is a Slow Process

Looking at the webpages of medical textbooks and cancer institutes, I learned that the liver has over 500 functions, all of them involved in the metabolism, the digestive process of vertebrates. The liver is divided into two lobes, a large one on the right, and a smaller one on the left. They consist of eight functionally independent segments. The liver is capable of regenerating itself from as little as a quarter, i.e. two segments, into a whole, fully functional organ.

Once I was aware of the complexity of this organ, I wanted to learn more about the possible cause of the illness since hepatitis, cirrhosis, and bilharzia had already been ruled out.

In anticipation of Cathy being cured of her illness, I began my search. Determining the origin of a problem can go a long way towards finding a solution and avoiding its recurrence. Or so I thought.

It turned out to be an arduous task because there is no list of possible causes of liver cancer or any other type of cancer besides the condemnations of an unhealthy lifestyle. The cause of the disease appears to be treated along the line of determining it does very little or nothing to cure it, prevent it from spreading, or avoid its recurrence – so, one might as well forget about looking for or even treating the cause.

My search felt like poking around in a dark tunnel with a short stick in the hope of hitting on something. The few hints I encountered all showed that once a patient has come down with cancer, it is pointless to investigate or treat the cause. There are practically no guidelines and hardly any established procedures to detect the cause, which is usually encountered only by happenstance. That is one of the biggest failures in the prevention and treatment of cancer for the following reasons.

Take aflatoxicosis, for example, the poisoning of food with aflatoxins, which I still suspect to this day was the cause of my wife's cancer.

Aflatoxin is a substance produced by the mould of the fungi *Aspergillus Flavus* and *A. Parasiticus* that grow in the soil all over the world. The poison is encountered in food crops for human consumption and livestock feed.

The food groups affected by this toxin are ranging from grain, fruit, nuts, vegetables and their derived products to milk and the meat of animals that feed on contaminated livestock fodder. When aflatoxicosis is encountered, every effort is undertaken to trace the origin of the disease in those countries that have a functioning food safety system, as in Europe for example. Once the source is found, the level of aflatoxin is measured.[1] Should it exceed the prescribed limit, the food will be destroyed by incineration. It is the only way to eradicate the toxic mould and avert the infection of not just hundreds but very likely thousands more people with aflatoxicosis.

About half a million people in China and several hundred thousand in India suffer aflatoxicosis every year and subsequently liver damage and in many cases cancer of the liver or kidneys and succumb to it. Should a patient be cured of the cancer caused by the ingestion of aflatoxin, an extremely rare occurrence, it is prudent for the doctor to explain the cause and advise the patient how to avoid a recurrence. Thus, it is only sensible to explain to patients why they should ascertain that their food is fresh and does not contain any signs of mould.

The same goes for the intake of headache or heartburn over-the-counter medications that were detected to contain carcinogens. Patients should be advised to refrain from taking these medicines to avoid a recurrence of their cancer.

Gaining no insights into the possible cause, I turned to the search for treatments and possible cures. A plethora of

---

[1] EU Maximum levels of aflatoxins (aflatoxins B1, B2, G1, G2 and M1) *Commission Regulation (EC) No 1881/2006 (https://eur-lex.europa.eu/legal-content/EN/TXT/PDF/?uri=CELEX: 02006R1881-20140701&from=EN)*

allegedly successful treatments and cures poured like slime out of the Internet. First in line were the homoeopaths and other quacks that praise their "natural" remedies with claims of having cured hundreds, even thousands of cancer patients. The worst of the lot were medical practitioners who claim to have scientific proof that the human body can heal itself of cancer tumours with happy thoughts and without any form of medical intervention. Although a positive frame of mind is helpful and supportive in a healing process, it is quackery to claim that positive thoughts and humming a mantra will heal terminal cancer patients of their Stage IV tumours that have metastasised all over the body.

Anecdotal evidence, which is not scientific proof, showed that there are indeed a few people who have "miraculously" recovered from cancer after various medical therapies failed to achieve the desired outcome. However, no matter how far a positive frame of mind enhances treatment, it is not the catalyst that helps to eradicate grapefruit-sized tumours suddenly and inexplicably. That claim belongs into the realm of fairy tales.

Also, those faith healers who claim their anecdotes to be scientific proof certainly know the difference between the back and front of a hundred dollar bill and how to rake in the dough. By the obverse of their claim they insinuate that the 9 million people who die from cancer every year essentially die as a result of negative thoughts and a lack of faith. One can only wonder if these quacks also belong to the faithful who kneel down beside their car and pray for a miracle to fix a flat tyre without any mechanical intervention as quite a few people especially in the bible belt of the USA are claimed to have been observed to do.

Next in line were pharma companies and their obedient servants, the medical journals. Almost every company involved in cancer research and the production of cancer medicine claims to have the one effective treatment for various types of cancer. Yet, it is a well-known fact that cytotoxic drugs in the best case only palliate, make a disease less severe without removing the cause, but do not cure cancer.

Besides leukaemia, skin and breast cancer, the majority of the other over 200 types of cancer were rarely if ever mentioned. The treatment of the liver was conspicuously absent, which was not surprising since further research revealed that cancer medications are metabolised by the liver and some of them even cause liver cancer.

Oh great! Was that the end of the road? For the time being, it was.

I had gained the insight that very little, if anything could be done to cure my wife's illness and I was cured of my faith in the "gods in white lab coats" and the pharma and biotech industries. But I would not give up my search for a cure.

Still, in the course over the next few weeks, I became what one could call a "medical atheist".

The Second and Decisive Misdiagnosis

Cathy had been given a blood test on the day of her devastating diagnosis to determine the level of bilirubin in her blood that was the cause of her jaundice.

Bilirubin is the orange-yellow pigment formed in the liver by the breakdown of haemoglobin. In the process of detoxification, synthesis, and production of biochemicals for the digestion of food and drink, the liver produces bile that is stored in the gall bladder, which concentrates and then releases it into the common bile duct that transports it into the small intestine where it helps with the digestion of fat.

In a healthy person the level of bilirubin is between 5 to 10 milligrams per decilitre (mg/dl). The test revealed that her bilirubin count was over 575mg/dl.

It was an indication of critical hyperbilirubinemia, a much higher than normal and potentially fatal level of bilirubin. It is caused by a large obstruction, in her case the tumour, blocking the hepatobiliary system, the arrangement of small ducts that secrete the bile from the liver into the hepatic ducts, the gall bladder, and the common bile duct.

It was decided that Cathy had to be hospitalised and I brought her to the Hepatology Ward of the Specialist Hospital of King Abdullah Medical City on Sunday, 22nd May 2016.

The ward is part of the most recent addition to the hospital complex, very clean, modern, and light with single hospital rooms.

A doctor, an expatriate from a Middle Eastern country, was introduced to us as the liver cancer specialist in charge of the team taking care of Cathy. He showed us the pictures of the CT scan. We saw the large tumour at the lower edge of the liver on the hepatic ducts or portal vein. There were some small secondary tumours in liver segments 3, 4, and 5.

Then the doctor pointed to a large growth at the top of the spleen. It was white with frayed edges that looked very

17

different from the tumour below the liver. He asserted that it was the original tumour, which had caused the cancer to metastasise into and onto the liver. Therefore, he concluded firmly, it was cancer of the spleen and a liver transplant or resection of the liver was out the question.

That was the misdiagnosis with fatal consequences for Cathy. Had I known then what I knew some time later, I should have insisted immediately and most forcefully on a biopsy of the growth on the spleen. It would have proved the doctor wrong and revealed that Cathy was a candidate for a resection or a liver transplant.

Unfortunately, at that moment I believed what that doctor told us. After all, he was a liver cancer specialist who was working with this illness every day and would know what he was talking about, right?

Wrong!

Not every doctor is a good doctor. Some will deliver their misdiagnosis, their mere conjecture with such aplomb that one doesn't even think of questioning their gobbledegook.

Please take note of this tragic development. Dare to question any medical practitioner's claim to have diagnosed a disease on the strength of having looked briefly at a picture without providing conclusive medical evidence. Then the diagnosis is not a diagnosis - it is merely full-throated blather that a charwoman, a public toilet attendant, or a drunk and lonely beachcomber without any medical training could have provided equally well!

It has to be questioned, discarded, and medical evidence demanded!

Emergency Measures

Upon Cathy's arrival in the hospital room, a young Saudi doctor turned up. He explained in detail the options of the emergency measures that had to be taken to lower the bilirubin count. For her benefit he clarified the function of the liver, the bile ducts, the gallbladder and that after its concentration the bile leaves through the common bile duct into the small intestine.

A catheter would be inserted into an hepatic bile duct and the attached bag would have to be emptied periodically. Once he clarified that the catheter would be a permanent fixture and the bag could fill up more than four times a day depending on the flow of bilirubin, we wanted to hear the other option. It was the insertion of flexible tubing, a stent into a hepatic duct, as well as a temporary catheter with a bag. Ultimately the catheter could be removed to facilitate the drainage of bilirubin into the small intestine. But, he contended right away, a stent would make a resection of the liver a bit difficult.

That was a strange statement. Hadn't the liver cancer specialist in charge of the team taking care of Cathy and presumably the Saudi doctor's superior just told us that a resection of the liver was out of the question?

When I asked him, he gave me an inscrutable smile and rolled his eyes in response. It was a very clear answer. Then he shook his head, chuckled, and muttered very quietly as if to assure that nobody outside the room could hear him, "Get a second opinion."

He was absolutely right, and I wish I had asked him there and then how and where to get one before he left the room. He was another example of the competent and dedicated young Saudi doctors with years of training in foreign countries who left me wondering why the hospitals in Saudi Arabia hire incompetent expatriate medics when they have hundreds of these talented medical practitioners of their own who often, as I should find out later, are desperate to find employment.

19

I encouraged Cathy to have a stent implanted and she was carted off for the insertion into the right hepatic duct for the drainage of the bilirubin. By late afternoon the deed was done, and the drainage bag filled up with a disgusting looking dark brown liquid.

Then we had another consultation with the doctor in charge. It was a sobering experience. He regurgitated what he had told us before: Cathy had cancer of the liver as a result of the spleen tumour's metastasis.

So, it wasn't cancer of the spleen any longer. That was a change of diagnosis I should have questioned right away and nailed him with it to his chair. He reiterated that the possibility of removing the cancer by resection or a liver transplant was impossible. He persisted in his diagnosis while admitting that it had not been determined with certainty if the large tumour below the liver was located either inside or outside the organ.

I asked him, if he was absolutely certain that the growth on the spleen was the main tumour and the disease would still be liver cancer if the large tumour underneath the liver were located outside the organ.

Like a broken record he repeated his assertion that the tumour on the spleen had metastasised to the liver and it was therefore liver cancer. Full stop! He proclaimed to be an expert in this matter and practically nothing could be done to get rid of the cancer except by resection, which in his opinion was out of the question.

That was shocking news. Recognising our consternation, he muttered on about treatments with transarterial radio embolisation, radiofrequency ablation, chemotherapy, and radiotherapy that could prevent the cancer from spreading and potentially destroy the tumours.

What now? In more or less the same breath he stated that there was no hope to get rid of the cancer but that one or the other of his suggested treatments could kill the tumours. Was he just trying to confuse us or was he raising false hopes to keep us calm? It was probably the latter because he concluded that the treatments would prolong the patient's life without stating for how long and declined to discuss the odds of the cancer cells getting killed by the treatments he suggested.

His consultation was once more a case of pure conjecture without providing any medical evidence.

I should have questioned his assertions and demanded evidence that could support his opinion. But heck, he was the doctor in charge of the team that was taking care of Cathy.

Who would want to argue with a cancer specialist that can provide proof of his knowledge and experience with more colourful certificates than he would need to wallpaper his toilet from ceiling to floor? And that's probably all his degrees, diplomas, and certificates are good for...

The Continued Search for the Cause

With a stent implant and the catheter taking care of Cathy's bilirubin, I intensified my search for the cause of her cancer and checked every possible source of information.

Just over two weeks earlier, Cathy had been as right as rain. I couldn't fathom how she could have been afflicted with cancer so suddenly and looked for acute causes.

That was a waste of time. I found out several days later that cancer is never an acute form of the illness that occurs suddenly within say a couple of months. It develops slowly and could have started a long time ago, quite possibly several years, even decades before a telltale sign results in the detection of malignant cancer tumours.

Cancer is not diagnosed when it is still in its infancy of Stage I or II but usually very late at the advanced Stage III or terminal Stage IV when it has metastasised. It makes the treatment with surgery and chemo- and radiotherapy so futile and is rarely crowned with a life extension and almost never with a cure.

There are many, yet only a finite number of possible causes. Since cirrhosis, hepatitis and bilharzia had been excluded, I thought that it had to have been something she ingested until I came across information about iron overload on the website of the Johns Hopkins Cancer Clinic in Baltimore, Maryland.[2]

It mentioned that people of Irish, Scottish, Welsh, Cornish, Breton, English and Scandinavian lineage are prone to suffer from haemochromatosis, i.e. iron overload. It was claimed that among the people of Irish origin about 10% of adults suffer iron overload, which can be cured quickly and easily when detected early. Yet, about 1% of men and women of Irish

---

[2] Hemochromatosis
(https://www.hopkinsmedicine.org/health/ conditions-and-diseases/ hemochromatosis)

22

origin still suffer liver cancer due to haemochromatosis and die as a result.

My wife was of Irish lineage and I had to find out if iron overload had caused her liver cancer. It took a while to find someone who could tell me if it had shown up in the numerous blood tests. Every doctor wanted to know why it was of any concern to me. So I had to explain to them that it could have been the cause of the cancer and if it was treated as recommended by the Johns Hopkins Cancer Centre it could prevent the recurrence of cancer. That was dismissed by these experts as irrelevant.

In the end it was a lab technician familiar with my wife's medical record who assured me that iron overload had not been detected. Thus, I scratched it off the list of possible causes and continued with my investigation.

Another potential cause of liver cancer is aflatoxicosis as mentioned earlier. It is important to note that the thousands of moulds used in and necessary for the production of consumable food such as cheese and bread as well as medicines like penicillin should not be confused with this toxic variety of fungus, aflatoxin.

Evidently only a tiny amount of aflatoxin entering the bloodstream after ingesting spoiled vegetables, fruits, baked goods, or contaminated dairy products and meat is enough to affect the liver and cause cancer. Larger amounts of aflatoxin can kill a person within three days.

Western European countries check all relevant food for aflatoxins but in Asia, Africa and Latin America these quite laborious and expensive tests are apparently conducted only as a pre-export requirement to avoid the agricultural goods being rejected and destroyed in the recipient countries. At least no other evidence could be found in the registers of the largest food exporting countries of these three continents that showed regular tests of all food groups particularly those destined for the national markets.

Saudi Arabia imports vast quantities of its food from these three continents. There is no official record of food imports being tested for aflatoxins in the kingdom. Consequently, it was fair to assume that aflatoxicosis could have been the cause of Cathy's liver cancer.

Since I prepared all the food we ate at home and made sure it was fresh and fit for consumption, it only could have happened as a result of Cathy eating lunch at the university cafeteria regularly since our arrival six years earlier.

Don't misunderstand that as an accusation of spoiled food being served in the restaurants of King Abdullah Medical City. Should it have happened there then the aflatoxin had entered the food chain much earlier in, for example, mouldy grain in its country of origin. The aflatoxin is not destroyed when grain is ground into flour or when the flour is ultimately used to bake bread. The only way to avoid aflatoxin entering the food chain, for humans and beasts alike, is to destroy the affected food by incineration.

I presented my findings to the doctor in charge and again got no response or any interest shown in the printed reports. When I questioned him about the possibility of aflatoxicosis being the cause of Cathy's illness, he didn't have a clue about the disease. This hepatological expert didn't even know what aflatoxin was, where it occurred, or that it caused liver cancer. Consequently, he was unwilling to discuss it, give me a minute of his time to consider it, or refer me to a doctor who knew something about it.

It goes to show that when you ask badass doctors about a disease that isn't of interest to them, even it is closely related to or could have been the cause of the illness they are treating - don't expect to get an answer!

Had the doctor taken the time to explain that the belated treatment of the cause of cancer doesn't change the outcome of the disease or its treatment, I could have accepted his reluctance to discuss it. But that didn't happen, did it?

The Ups and Downs of Treatment

Daily visits and spending as much time with Cathy as possible and as long as the hospital permitted me to stay helped to keep up her spirits and let her forget for brief moments the utter devastation we both felt.

Cathy started to look and feel better since the drainage of the bilirubin had shown some effect. But the daily blood tests revealed that the count had stalled at approximately 275 mg/dl, a still very critical level.

It had become apparent that also the left hepatic bile duct had to have a stent inserted to improve the flow of bile.

Thus, it was decided on Thursday, 26th May 2016, to replace the stent in the right hepatic bile duct with a slightly larger one and to insert a second stent and a catheter into the left hepatic duct as well. It was hoped to finally lower the bilirubin count to the level of less than 50mg/dl, which was necessary to start any of the treatments that were supposed to tackle the cancer cells.

The replacement of the right hepatic duct stent was done quickly but the insertion of a stent into the left hepatic duct was easier said than done.

A stent of the appropriate size could not be found in the hospital. Other hospitals didn't have it either. Manufacturers in California and France were contacted. They could deliver it but with an order to be placed, the handling and shipping, and the import bureaucracy, it would take a week to ten days to arrive. That was considered too long a waiting period in this critical situation and turned out to be a hiccup with potentially crippling consequences for the procedures that had been suggested.

It was decided to insert at catheter. With the drainage tubes in place, Cathy had two bags dangling off her sides. They filled up rapidly with a flow of the bile that was now assumed to be sufficient to bring the bilirubin count down.

Right after this intervention five different doctors felt obliged to consult Cathy. The optimists among them tried to convince us that everything was under control and that Cathy would soon be healthy again. The pessimists in contrast told us that everything possible had been done and that there was no hope for a cure. The only point of agreement among the optimists and pessimists was the bilirubin count. It had to be brought down to below 50mg/dl before tackling the tumours with ablation or embolisation.

The doctors talked a lot, yet not one of them was taking charge for procedures and treatment. The contradiction of statements confused us and resulted in us not taking any of them seriously any longer.

Once the flood of consultations ebbed away over the next couple of days, we were kept in the dark about Cathy's actual status and felt shunted aside.

I talked to the Patient Relations Officer about the doctors' obvious prejudice (because we are not Muslims) as well as their failure to keep Cathy in a positive frame of mind with procedural updates. It bore no results.

We did not expect to get help or a clear answer with the Muslims' holy month of Ramadan slated to start on 7th June 2016.

Quite a few members of the hospital staff had already reduced their work schedule, as is the norm in Saudi Arabia during Ramadan, or they had gone on vacation in some unholy overseas country where they could enjoy a roasted pork hock and quaff a big jug of beer.

Cathy and I had observed several traditionally dressed Arabs engaged in such impious activity during a visit to a restaurant in Munich a couple of years earlier.

First Mention of 'Palliative Care'

What had appeared to be a straightforward path of the next steps to be taken became all muddled when the doctor in charge visited on Thursday, 2nd June 2016 to inform us that neither ablation nor embolisation could be performed for dubious reasons and no other therapy would be effective.

It became obvious that he wanted to wash his hands of any further responsibility for Cathy's treatment and tried to slough her off when he laconically stated that the Oncology Ward would cure her with palliative care.

His haughty disdain for Cathy and me had already set my teeth on edge every time he talked to us on previous occasions but this time he had gone too far.

Stating that none of the therapies would be effective and that the Oncology Ward could take care of a cure was a contradiction because he described palliative care as the application of a therapy the oncologist deemed appropriate and effective for a cure. But since he had stated that none would show any effect what was the point? Was he trying to tell us that Cathy had only a few more days to live?

I blew my top and tore into him with a barrage of questions. Did he know that the term 'palliative' is derived from the Latin verb *'palliare'*, which means 'to cloak, to cover up'?

What was he trying to cover up, I asked him - his inability to treat cancer, his incompetence, or was he quite possibly not even a bona fide doctor?

He stormed out of the room. I went after him and demanded a copy of the entire medical record upon which his diagnosis was based.

An administrator and the head nurse joined the confrontation and denied me the right to obtain the medical record. It was fortunate that at this moment the doctor of the Oncology Ward who was supposed to take care of Cathy came for a visit in the company of a Saudi friend of mine. They intervened pointing out that every patient has the right to obtain the medical records for a second opinion. Grudgingly the administrator got off her high horse and gave me permission to get the entire medical record in digital format on a disc. She chose this soft copy, as I found out once I had received it, because the data can be accessed only with a special computer program available exclusively to hospitals.

The oncologist's visit had a calming effect on Cathy and me. His manners were impeccable when he explained the various options he would pursue to deal with the cancer. But he warned also that any treatment would take between four to six weeks to show any noticeable effect. He encouraged me as well to get a second opinion and gave us hope that not everything was lost.

My Saudi friend told me afterwards that he had contacts with doctors at the King Feisal Specialist Hospital in Riyadh. He would call them to see if they could provide a second opinion. Furthermore, he assured me to speak with the head of the Hepatology Ward and have the doctor in charge of Cathy's team taken off her case.

Two days later this came to pass. Sadly, the guy who replaced him, yet another expatriate doctor of Middle Eastern origin, was just another bigmouth with the bedside manner of a boar in heat and the attention span of a fruit fly, as we should find out over the next few days.

That night back home I established contact with medical groups in France, Germany and England to get their opinion about treatment of liver cancer. The responses were not very encouraging. They stated in unison that the survival time of a patient with liver cancer was between six months and two years unless the cancer was surgically removed, which did not exclude a recurrence of the cancer. However, a conclusive answer could only be given after a review of the CT scans and all of them were very eager to help and awaited a copy of the medical record.

This stands in stark contrast to the Canadian Cancer Society's high-handed response. It stated bluntly that it refuses to provide a second opinion to anyone outside of Canada and advised to rely on local cancer specialists wherever the patient happens to be regardless of the patient being a Canadian citizen or not.

I informed Cathy's sister in Canada about our situation and tried to circumnavigate the Canadian Cancer Society's callous obstinacy by asking her to take a copy of the medical record to a local cancer centre and request a second opinion.

That did not work either, as we should find out a few days later. It was a projection of what should await us in Canada after our return.

A Second Opinion and Hope at Last

The soft copy of the medical record on disc was ready for pick-up at the record centre on Sunday, 4ᵗʰ June 2016. The young lady in charge did not object to my request for a second disc as a result of our chat about her mother who suffered from cancer.

I advised her to avoid Canada like the pest based on the response I had received from the Canadian Cancer Society and recommended to contact the Charité Hospital in Berlin, Germany, that appeared to specialise in the treatment of her mother's cancer - glioblastoma. Many months later I learned that her mother had been treated successfully in Berlin and was recuperating in Saudi Arabia.

My Saudi friend informed me that he had contacted a friend of his, a doctor at the King Feisal Specialist Hospital and gave me his phone number. I called and arranged an appointment for Tuesday, 7ᵗʰ June 2016. I was a bit concerned about the date because it was the first day of Ramadan when all Muslims, including doctors and nurses have a fifty percent reduced work schedule and everything comes to a virtual standstill. But the doctor assured me that I would be given the requested second opinion - no ifs or buts.

The oncologist visited Cathy again on Monday, 6ᵗʰ June 2016, and gave her a thorough exam. He expressed his concern about the bilirubin count still above 100mg/dl and stated that it had to come down to below 50mg/dl before he could undertake a treatment with embolisation, i.e. shrinking the tumours, or killing them with radiotherapy.

He assured her as well that the essential treatment with antibiotics and the draining of bilirubin would continue even during Ramadan. He wanted to have the catheters and bags removed and urged his colleagues in the Hepatology Ward to insert the second stent.

He was informed that the stent ordered from France was scheduled to arrive on Thursday next. In summary he sounded very positive about successfully treating the cancer and welcomed the news about me going to obtain a second opinion from another cancer specialist.

The big day that would bring some clarity into the cancer diagnosis or confirm doom and gloom had arrived at last. In the morning of Tuesday, 7th June 2016, and after parking the car in a no-stopping zone of the endless construction site of the King Feisal Hospital, I rushed into the lobby clutching the disc that contained the pictures of the CT scan.

Dr. Khaled received me with open arms and took me to a room full of computer display terminals. His colleague, Dr. Mohammed who was familiar with the operation of the computer system and the specialised software for viewing the CT scan popped the disc into the drive and looked at the pictures. He shook his head, took out the disc, waved it about, and gave me a look that asked, "W.t.f. is this?"

Briefly I worried that these doctors could not provide a second opinion but then I was complimented into another darkened room with only one but humongous display terminal. They switched on the computer and Dr. Mohammed explained that it was a three-dimensional colour display system that would allow them to view the pictures in detail that the other black and white displays, which were also used at the King Abdullah Hospital, did not facilitate.

The two doctors, both of them having served their internship in Canada, popped the disc into the computer and studied the CT scan pictures. They took their time and were very meticulous to get a view of the tumours from all possible angles. I stood behind them and watched.

They discussed among them what they saw and finally turned to me with the question what path of action the doctors at the King Abdullah Hospital had recommended.

I told them that the initially mentioned surgery had been abandoned and that the oncologist appointed to continue the treatment seemed eager to try embolisation as well as chemo-

and radiotherapy. Also, a second stent was to be inserted into the right hepatic duct to increase the discharge of bilirubin. So far the only firm conclusion had been that a resection of the liver, a lobectomy was out of the question because the cancer had metastasised from the spleen onto the liver.

Both doctors looked at me in disbelief and then gave me their verdict while pointing at the screen display to underscore what they told me. First of all, they assured me that segments six and seven of the liver were not affected by the cancer. They did not detect a single spot that would have indicated a metastasis on either one of these segments, which is the precondition for a possible surgical intervention, a resection of the liver.

Then they expressed their doubts that the growth on the spleen was actually a cancer tumour. It looked nothing like the large cancer tumour underneath the liver and was probably benign, which meant that they agreed with the Saudi general practitioner at King Abdullah Hospital who had assumed it to be benign. However, a biopsy would have to confirm it and should be done as soon as possible.

Yet, independent of the results of the biopsy that would determine if the growth on the spleen was benign or not, they stated clearly and succinctly that the large cancer tumour was not inside or on the liver. It was outside of the organ but due to the angles of the pictures they could not ascertain that it was on a bile duct below the hilum where the two bile ducts join, the hepatic artery, or the portal vein.

They assured me it was extrahepatic and specifically distal cholangiocarcinoma, commonly known as bile duct cancer that had metastasised to the liver. That type of cancer requires a different treatment and medication than liver cancer.

Liver cancer tumours are treated with a medication called Nexavar that is supposed to stop the tumours' blood supply and hopefully lead to their eventual apoptosis. Bile duct cancer on the other hand should be treated with the drugs

Cisplatin or Gemcitabine that cause the tumours to shrink or at least stop their growth and metastasis.

They concluded that their colleagues at the King Abdullah Hospital were wrong with their diagnosis of liver cancer because even when bile duct cancer metastasises to the liver it is still bile duct cancer. They explained that there are three types of cholangiocarcinoma: intrahepatic, the rarest form that occurs on the bile ducts inside the liver, perihilar on the hilum where the two major bile ducts join just below the liver, and distal below the hilum but above the cystic duct that leads to the gall bladder.

Both perihilar and distal bile duct cancer are extrahepatic, meaning they occur outside the liver. In all cases the tumour blocks the bile ducts and the flow of the bile, which resulted in Cathy's jaundice that had led to the cancer diagnosis.

Then they broached the subject of the insertion of stents to bring down the bilirubin count to well below 50mg/dl. The insertion of hepatic duct stents should only be considered when the other options of using catheters and administering bilirubin-binding medication have been proven to be fruitless. The presence of stents in the hepatic ducts makes a surgical intervention and resection of the liver quite difficult although not impossible.

However, they stated that Cathy was a good candidate for surgery. They suggested to have her hospitalised at the King Feisal Specialist Hospital where the resection could be done.

They explained that a specialist surgeon from overseas would arrive within six weeks. He could clean up the entire mess by resecting the liver and removing the growth on the spleen. Six to eight weeks after the operation the liver would have regenerated itself and Cathy would be free of cancer and as healthy as she had been before cancer struck.

That was the good news I had hoped to hear. I was elated until we talked about the cost of hospitalising Cathy at the King Feisal Specialist Hospital.

The doctors were not quite sure how much it would cost. It would depend on the nationality of the surgeon. An American surgeon, although not any better than his Australian or European counterparts, would probably charge almost double the amount of his peers. But no matter what the amount of the bill would be, it would have to be paid 'cash on the barrelhead' by the health insurance or privately.

That put a damper on my elation, but I rushed back to bring Cathy the good news. We were happy and very hopeful that her ordeal could be over in less than two months.

And then Cathy said the fateful words: "It sounds almost too good to be true."

When Something Sounds Too Good to be True...

... it usually is too good to be true as we should find out quickly. It was not a case of the doctors at the King Feisal Specialist Hospital having changed their mind. No, their offer stood firmly, but at the King Abdullah Hospital things turned against us.

I consulted the representative of the National Guard Health Insurance to learn if the costs of surgery at the King Feisal Specialist Hospital would be covered.

The man was a kind old doctor whose permanent facial expression was probably a reflection of all the suffering he had seen in his lifetime.

Patiently he explained the confusing situation of "universal" health care in Saudi Arabia. It is and it is not universal at the same time. Every employer is compelled by law to provide health care insurance to every employee free of charge. In so far the health care is universal. But health care insurance is provided by several different companies and each company covers only a limited number of doctors and hospitals under its schemes.

The King Feisal Specialist Hospital is a private hospital and not covered by the health insurance of the National Guard, said the doctor. The only option was to have Cathy treated as a private patient. A quick telephone inquiry informed the doctor and me that the suggested surgery and a stay of at least two weeks in the hospital would cost about $250,000 and probably more than that. That was an amount Cathy and I couldn't afford and there was no way to raise it privately, especially as we were expatriates. Philanthropy is reserved for Saudi citizens and preferably Sunni Muslims of the Wahhabi persuasion, either of which did not and does not apply to us.

That blow below the belt was not all that day. Upon my return to Cathy the doctor who had misdiagnosed the growth on her spleen had suddenly been put in charge again and was giving his usual cock and bull twaddle.

35

I confronted him with the second opinion diagnosis, demanded a biopsy of the growth on the spleen as well as conclusive medical evidence to support his diagnosis.

He rejected the second opinion out of hand claiming to know more about cancer than the two medical peers he had never met and didn't know. Also, a biopsy of the growth was not necessary because he had recognised that growth as cancer. Finally, he declared a referral to the King Feisal Hospital unnecessary because his team was doing everything that could be done for Cathy.

Having become quite impatient listening to him sounding off, I asked him calmly how many patients in his care die every year and if there were any survivors.

In response he shouted something in Arabic, probably a verbal shoe thrown in my direction, the ultimate insult in the Middle East, and stormed out - never to be seen again by us.

I learned a bit later that he had demanded to be released of his duty of being in charge of the team caring for this patient on account of her obnoxious husband. I took that as a compliment and was happy to be rid of him.

Rounding out the day was a little bit of good news. One of the doctors of the Hepatology Ward had found by sheer coincidence a stent in his desk that was the correct size for insertion into the right hepatic duct of Cathy's liver.

Wonders will never cease, will they?

Cathy was carted off and the stent was inserted. When she was returned to her room, the two bags filled up. Nurses were put on standby to change the bags and I went home with relative peace of mind that the bilirubin count would be brought down to below the critical level of 50mg/dl.

And onto a Slippery Slope We Went

Despite the bilirubin count coming down steadily to clear the path for the planned treatment, many questions remained especially concerning the tumours. Will they shrink or can they be eradicated and leave only scar tissue?

It appeared to be an almost irrelevant question because the doctors seemed to be of the opinion that once you have cancer, it will never go away and despite killing the existing tumours, the cancer will recur.

Also, I still had the question why the cause or origin of Cathy's cancer was not investigated or even considered in view of any future treatment. That question was never answered. It seemed the doctors were scared of opening a Pandora's box of food safety in Saudi Arabia because every aspect pointed to aflatoxin poisoning.

As a result of my research, I had garnered information about hepatocellular carcinoma and cholangiocarcinoma as well as various medications and different approaches to the surgical removal of liver cancer tumours.

The pharmaceutical companies from around the world claim, of course, that their medications can do wonders battling various types of cancer. But liver or bile duct cancer never featured in their claims and even specialist hospitals of world renown didn't list these two types on their pages of information about different cancers.

What struck me as peculiar was the information about liver cancer surgery in Canada. Many times I came across reports of a liver transplant performed on a cancer patient diagnosed with cirrhosis of the liver or hepatitis but not when these two ailments were not detected, as was the case with my wife.

What was the reason? Were the doctors in cahoots with alcoholics and careless people who ignored warnings about picking up hepatitis? Not finding answers, I questioned the doctors but didn't get any clarifications.

A further aspect of note was the difference of opinion between the team of doctors supposedly treating Cathy and the oncologist as well as Dr. Khaled and Dr. Mohammed. The team claimed that a resection of the liver was 'impossible' once the stents were inserted even if the tumours had been shrunk to a small operable size.

Contrary to that claim, the latter three doctors stated that a resection is not impossible but a bit complicated. Such resection could very well be done by a specialist surgeon who would take the 'aggressive' approach of a lobectomy, remove the largest part of the liver except Segments VI and VII, and replace the damaged bile ducts with suitable material, either man-made or natural.

The difference of opinion had to be expected, though. Cancer treatment is not an issue of agreement and compliance with the view of only one expert.

On Thursday, 16th June 2016, a crucial blood test was on Cathy's agenda. Her bilirubin count had already come down to 65mg/dl on her last test and it was anticipated that it would be down to below 50mg/dl. Should that be the case (and everybody kept their fingers crossed) then the drain tubes and catheter bags would be removed, and she could get ready to go home.

Amazingly the result of the latest blood test was announced only two hours later. The news travelled fast, and we were again confronted by the doctor with the bedside manner of a boar in heat who had replaced the loudmouth.

He disregarded my request for a biopsy of the growth on the spleen insisting in perfect harmony with the loudmouth's first assertion that the growth on the spleen was the primary cancer tumour. A resection or a liver transplant was therefore out of the question and hence, Cathy had to leave the Hepatology Ward where liver surgery could have been performed. Since her bilirubin count had come down to below the acceptable level of 50mg/dl, he declared her fit to be treated as an outpatient in the Oncology Ward for palliative care, where she would be cured.

What? She would be cured? Was the doctor joking? I gobsmacked him with the oncologist's statements about him trying to achieve the best possible outcome of shrinking the tumours and the treatment would only palliate the symptoms by making them less severe without removing the cause.

Rarely have I seen a doctor with a more stupid expression on his face when I challenged him to explain what he meant by Cathy being 'cured' and demanded what he understood the term 'palliative care' to mean. Like his predecessor he had no clue that it is an end of life treatment of simply drowning the cancer pain in a flood of toxic medicines and morphine or fentanyl that will not have any curative effect when the patient is considered incurable and expected to die. So, what gave him the idea that Cathy would be cured?

He left and shouted in the hallway to have Cathy removed within the hour. Fortunately, one of his colleagues, again one of the young Saudi doctors, had the sense to have the two drainages removed late in the afternoon. Once that was done, he came back and told us to ignore that doctor. He explained that the head of the Hepatology Ward was out of the country, which caused the battle between expatriate and Saudi doctors. Some expatriates with seniority asserted to be at the helm and claimed to be in charge. The doctor let Cathy stay for the night since we had not received referral papers and the Oncology Ward was closed for the day.

The following morning a different doctor explained the procedure lying ahead for Cathy. I had no objection to pack up her stuff and take her home. But there was still the issue of the guide wires for the drainage tubes sticking out of her sides. We were not going to leave the ward until they had been removed. Bedlam ensued.

Midday prayer time approached, and I had left Cathy at the reception desk while I was desperately looking for a medic who could remove the wires. I was shouted at by the staff to get out. They were desperate to get up on the roof for a smoke and a drink, which is strictly prohibited during Ramadan in the daytime. But since the Matawa, the religious police didn't have helicopters it was safe to indulge in some sinful activity on the roof of that six-storey building.

Then I heard Cathy scream and saw the doctor in charge trying to drag her physically out of the ward and lock the door. I rushed in between them and knocked his hand off her arm. I threatened to call the police to have him arrested and thrown in prison. In Saudi Arabia it is forbidden for a man to touch a woman outside of family and marriage bond, even for a doctor, except for a medical exam.

A nurse claimed that all operating theatres were closed for the day. I told her that we would stay until the wires had been removed and she should find somebody to do that.

A medic turned up expressing his disgust about nobody wanting to resolve the issue and made that abundantly clear to his colleagues. He found a storage room where he could do the good deed. We moved all the cluttered stuff into the hallway, cleaned an exam table, and Cathy clambered up. Within fifteen minutes the wires had been removed and we were on our way home after thanking the medic for his initiative.

Our cat Sparky gave us a rousing feline welcome rubbing up against Cathy's legs and with a big smile. Some people say that cats don't smile. I beg to differ. One has to look at the expression of their eyes, not a showing of teeth and a lolling tongue as canine friends and companions do.

We settled in and Cathy enjoyed her favourite special meal I had made although she still could hardly taste anything. Good news was that her olfactory sense was almost entirely restored.

Palliative Care - The First

The following days we were busy with the bureaucracy of registering Cathy in the Oncology Ward and radiotherapy. There was also the requirement for Cathy to speak to her superior and the director of her college.

Her superior gave her a warm welcome and said that she would do everything in her power to accommodate her needs and assure that she could keep her job since she was a highly valued member of the faculty.

Cold water was poured over these promises by the director, an oncologist, or so he claimed, an hour later. He was very blunt, gave Cathy short shrift, and said that her contract would not be renewed and the automatic extension was cancelled.

If and when she was cured of the cancer, she could always reapply for a contract and he would consider it cautiously. But all her promotions over the past six years would be null and void and the best she could expect was a contract with a lengthy trial period at the beginner's salary.

Then he added his most idiotic suggestion because her contract ended on 15th October. He declared that we had to go on the legally decreed annual four-week vacation, return to Riyadh to dissolve our household, and then leave for good.

He wouldn't listen to Cathy's much more sensible request of moving the vacation period to the end of her contract and the termination date four weeks forward, so we could leave in the middle of September. That would probably have involved some work for him and therefore he couldn't possibly entertain such a request.

Insisting on us having to stick to his schedule, he created additional stress for Cathy that contributed to a worsening of her condition. Instead of having to take only one fourteen-hour flight, he forced us to take three with all the uncertainty that is normal when one has to change planes halfway through the flight.

We met the oncologist in charge of palliative care when he explained the schedule for the envisaged treatment. I will hold him in high regard for taking his time to calmly explain to us the ramifications of the cancer therapy and his ability to put Cathy's mind at rest.

But when I mentioned the second opinion I had obtained from King Feisal Hospital and the firm diagnosis of bile duct cancer that would require a different medication than liver cancer, he shrugged and declared that he had to stick to the diagnosis of the Hepatology Ward.

We looked at the CT scan pictures on his computer that had a relatively small 13-inch screen. He pointed at the number of tumours on the liver. The display was very blurry. He could not enlarge the image sufficiently to have a better view of the tumour underneath the liver. In conclusion he said, "Let us proceed on the path recommended by the doctor of the Hepatology Ward."

Thus, the misdiagnosis of the alleged hepatologists became firmly established and the doctors in Canada who continued treatment were also happy to abide by it.

Four sessions of radiotherapy were prescribed as well as the chemotherapy drug Nexavar that Cathy obtained free of charge at the hospital's pharmacy. The side effects of the chemotherapy were mentioned, and some medications prescribed that were supposed to alleviate these effects.

The oncologist was very calm and kind and obviously tried to assuage Cathy's fears. Yet he could not provide any information of the chances of a positive outcome. His palliative care could be summarised along the line, "Let's give this a try and see what happens."

Over the next five days, Cathy received the first batch of radiotherapy and she took the chemotherapy drug as prescribed. In the evening of the second day the drug's side effects hit her hard. Her legs had started to swell up enormously, she started to itch intensely all over, and when she took a shower her hair was falling out considerably. I suggested not taking the chemo drug until the next appointment with the oncologist. That was two days to go.

The drug-free days helped a bit. The itching stopped almost entirely, her hair stopped falling out, and the swelling of her legs went down. But now Cathy was really scared that she could not get rid of her cancer with these drugs or any other therapy.

The oncologist suggested to take half the recommended dosage of Nexavar but insisted that she had to continue with the regimen to starve the tumours of their blood supply.

And so it continued with the side effects returning as soon as Cathy took as little as a quarter of the prescribed drug dosage. When she decided to take it only every second day, it didn't help either.

Despite the problems with the chemotherapy drug, the oncologist declared Cathy fit to travel before we left on our "vacation".

We requested a referral notice for the purpose of receiving a second opinion in Canada and learned that international referrals are not possible.

Instead he wrote an extensive medical report and I picked up the biopsy medical blocks. These blocks are 'unstained' glass slides for viewing under a microscope that provide a clear picture of how the doctors in Riyadh arrived at their cancer diagnosis.

The oncologist wished us a safe trip and assured us that the results of the radiotherapy would be available after our return.

"Fun and Games" in Canada

We departed Riyadh on 14th July at 1:00 am local time, arrived in Montreal the same day around noon, and on we went to our home turf, Ottawa.

The next morning Cathy called the Cancer Centre of the Ottawa General Hospital and requested an appointment with an oncologist for a review of the medical report and a second opinion. She was asked by the woman of the cancer ward answering her call where and when the report had been issued. Cathy stated that it was written by her oncologist in Saudi Arabia two days prior.

She was told that the report had to be translated which would take from four to six weeks.

Cathy told her that the report was written in impeccable English. The woman repeated like an automaton that it had to be translated. Into what language did it have to be translated? Hindi? Swahili? Chinese? It was written in error-free English by a medical professional, an oncologist!

Well, said that nauseating woman, then it had to be approved by a government certified translator and hung up.

Welcome to Canada's health care system!

Another call to the general inquiry desk yielded the result that Cathy only needed a referral from her Canadian family doctor to get an appointment with an oncologist.

A family doctor? Was that woman joking? There is such a shortage of general practitioners in Canada that some communities have organised a lottery to determine the winner who can get an appointment with the local GP!

This is to an extent due to what one could call Canadian arrogance of thinking that Canadian trained medics are better than any other medic. At present there are among the immigrants many skilled, highly educated and experienced general practitioners, specialists including oncologists, nurse practitioners, and nurses. Unfortunately, nobody knows the exact number of how many of those medics are in Canada. But every one of them is prohibited from working in the field of their education and experience until they have jumped through all the bureaucratic hoops of having obtained their basic education equivalence certificates, gone through Canadian education courses in their professional field of specialisation for which they have to pay, and taken and passed all the tests to certify their Canadian education.

So, during a visit to Canadian shores don't be surprised when the guy driving a taxi turns out to be a neurosurgeon or the woman mopping tables in a saloon is an oncologist.

Even highly qualified and specialised Canadian citizens who happen to have obtained their training and certification outside of Canada and are valued in their country of residence for their skills and expertise will run into the same roadblock if they want to come "home". They may be invited to participate in international conferences, some of them as keynote speakers, where they are lauded and praised by the media and bureaucrats alike as ambassadors of Canadian skill and goodwill. But coming back and working in their home country is a "No-No". Any educational certificate obtained outside of Canada is not worth the paper it is printed on once in Canada as Cathy and I had already found out with our degrees from Australia and England.

Medical staff is probably in short supply in most countries. What Canada could do to alleviate its shortage of medics would be to provide free of charge all tests that are required to establish the immigration applicants' level of skill and expertise before they enter their country of choice. Once the immigrants have arrived at their destination, they would be welcomed, treated like any nationally educated peer, and could start their work immediately.

In the end Cathy was informed that any walk-in clinic could also issue a referral. After several tries we found one that was open. The doctor gave her a somewhat strange exam. He was one of those doctors who had jumped through all the hoops, taken all the courses and exams, and was now a "qualified Canadian" general practitioner.

I wondered if he was illiterate and couldn't read the medical report or didn't want to take the time. He was rushing around metaphorically with his hair on fire, asked Cathy to lie on the exam table, and poked into her abdomen. He noticed a lump and asked what that was. I told him that it was probably the large cancer tumour and queried if he was trying to burst it. He said that he would write the referral and send it off right away. Cathy could expect a call in a day or two for an appointment at a cancer clinic.

When she had not received the confirmation for an appointment from the hospital, she called the walk-in clinic. They looked into the problem and told Cathy that the doctor had faxed the referral to an alternative treatment clinic that offered to pump lemon juice into her veins as a sure-fire cure for her cancer. That was not what Cathy wanted or needed and requested the referral to be sent to the Cancer Ward of the Ottawa Hospital. She was assured that it would be done.

We didn't get a call from the hospital and Cathy was discouraged to phone the cancer clinic again on account of her previous experience. Instead she had a long telephone conversation with her good friend Alison who offered to help. We decided to leave Ottawa and drove to the area northwest of Toronto where the friend resides.

After long and sometimes quite tearful discussions about what was best to do, Alison wheedled an appointment out of a clinic near her residence and the doctor wrote a referral to a hospital with a cancer ward some 80km away.

In the meantime I had come across a TV-documentary about D,L-methadone and the successful treatment of cancer patients in Germany. I followed up with more research and found a number of encouraging reports.[3] I showed Cathy the reports and she became hopeful that we would find a cure. But before we could contemplate a stopover in Germany, we had the appointment in the hospital.

It turned out to be another disappointment although the nurse practitioner was very helpful and listened to what we had to say. She inquired about secondary symptoms like abdominal pain and any sleep or eating problems. She was obviously quite concerned and read the medical report intently before she went ahead and called the resident oncologist for the consultation.

The doctor came in and plunked himself down. One arm dangling over the backrest and manspreading, he would have made a good impression as an intermission clown.

He flipped through the report without reading it and then mouthed off in his lilting accent while looking out of the window that everything that could be done for Cathy had been done. He got up and left. Consultation over.

The nurse practitioner's facial expression was a mix of disappointment and disgust. She had another chat with us in a very quiet and apologetic tone but made clear that there was nothing else she could do besides prescribing some mild opioid that would be a pain relief in case it was needed.

That was the end of that road. Cathy and I did more research for cancer treatments in Canada and came across reports about cryosurgery, NanoKnife treatments, and liver surgery.[4]

Cathy contacted the NanoKnife specialist and sent him a CD of the medical record so he could see the CT scan pictures.

---

[3] Fighting cancer with methadone - making chemotherapy more powerful, *18th Aug. 2016*
(*http://www.dw.com/en/fighting-cancer-with-methadone-making-chemotherapy-more-powerful/a-19482264*)
[4] Toronto surgeon redefines 'hopeless' cancer cases, *24th Feb. 2012*
(*Megan Ogilvie, Health Reporter, Toronto Star*)

A few days later he responded with the apology that he could not treat her cancer because the prime tumour *underneath* the liver was already too large.

In retrospect, it was very telling that the NanoKnife specialist referred to the prime tumour being underneath the liver, meaning that he shared the opinion of it being bile duct cancer, which would explain why he could not apply the NanoKnife technology that is designed especially for the apoptosis of small tumours on the liver. The question that arose was why none of the other specialists looking at the same CT scan pictures did not come to his conclusion of it being bile duct cancer.

And on we went to Canada's foremost cancer research and treatment hospital in Toronto. After a bit of haggling we got a pre-exam consultation with a young doctor. He was the polar opposite to the oncologist we had seen a few days earlier. Not only did he read the medical report, but also he listened to us most courteously and took my comment about the bile duct cancer diagnosis of his peers at the King Feisal Hospital into consideration.

He was very encouraging and gave us hope that we were in good hands. In regard to the bile duct cancer second opinion diagnosis he stated that Cathy would have to have another CT scan to get a clear picture of the actual type of cancer that would have to be followed up with the appropriate therapy.

Next we saw a radiologist who had a look at the CT scan from Riyadh. She was not impressed by the quality and arranged a scan in the hospital on the same day.

An appointment for a few days later was arranged with the surgeon who had developed a new approach to resecting a liver.

The end of our "vacation" was getting closer and in light of some delays with the consultations in Toronto, I called our travel agent in Riyadh and had him move our return flight by a couple of weeks to 1st September. He sent us the e-tickets

48

and we were all set for our flight. An explicit two-hour stopover only in Frankfurt was putting a crimp in any plan we had for a short stay in Germany to learn more about D,L-methadone and have Cathy undergo that treatment - but we had no choice.

During the following two weeks we undertook three more trips to Toronto for consultation with the radiologist and the surgeon.

Cathy was surprised that I could drive on those days the return trip of about a thousand kilometres (620 miles) in one day from very early morning until late at night without falling asleep at the wheel. What kept me awake and agitated was my concern for her and also the somewhat discouraging news we received from the radiologist as well as the surgeon's inconclusive assessments of her condition. We were told that in the relatively short time span of only six weeks a concrete diagnosis of her actual cancer, the appropriate treatment, a specific therapy, or a prognosis could not be provided. We believed it, were not cognisant of our trip to Canada having been a complete and utter waste of time, and already looked forward to our return in the middle of October.

In hindsight I concluded that we should have gone to Cuba for prompt and affordable treatment to stop the growth and spread of the cancer and possibly a lobectomy. But I had not been aware of the medical service provided in that Caribbean country. I only found out about it when it was too late - far too late.

So, the day approached when we took our flight back to Riyadh that started with a long drive to the Montreal airport in a rental car with expired license plates.

Once More Back "Home"

The following six weeks were a mad rush between hospital visits, dissolving our household that had been our home for six years, visits to the veterinarian to get an international vaccination certificate akin to a passport for Sparky, and deciding what to pack. It involved also finding an airline that would allow us to take Sparky with us in the passenger cabin. Lufthansa was the most obliging airline with a clear outline in this matter, but we had to obtain a ticket for our cat, which was all right and not too expensive.

The oncologist at the King Abdullah Hospital was not surprised about the outcome of our consultations in Canada. He didn't say anything negative or derogatory, but his facial expression said, "I didn't expect anything else."

He didn't have any good news either. The radiotherapy had not resulted in any shrinkage or apoptosis of the cancer tumours.

When I asked him about treatment with Cisplatin or Gemcitabine for bile duct cancer, he waved my question off and stated once more that he had to abide by the diagnosis of his colleagues in the Hepatology Ward. They insisted once more that it was cancer of the spleen that had metastasised to the liver and therefore liver cancer.

It was infuriating to hear such nonsense. Then he admitted that the diagnosis of bile duct cancer was probably correct, but he couldn't start a therapy because the two drugs for that type of cancer were not available at the King Abdullah Hospital at that time. So, he continued the treatment of liver cancer on the principle of hope but more than likely in full knowledge of it being futile.

Taking quite vigorous walks with Cathy late at night when the mild temperatures permitted such an exercise helped her a bit. She appeared to get better and it raised my hopes that the next visits to the oncologist would show some improvement. But the next CT scans put an end to that hope.

50

There was not a sign that the prescribed therapies showed any, not even the slightest advance or positive development.

Almost furiously I searched for different treatments and again came across the whole spectrum of quacks with their unproven remedies.

What was surprising were some reports about natives of Canada and Russia allegedly preventing the occurrence and even the healing of cancer with the ingestion of an infusion of the Smooth Sumac as well as small amounts of the tree fungus Chaga that is encountered in the far north of their respective countries. All very interesting but it wouldn't help Cathy.

What I wanted to find was a treatment that would get rid of her cancer by apoptosis of the tumours. And the only one I found was the little success story of the racemic aqueous solution D,L-methadone.

There were a number of detailed scientific reports documenting every step of the medication's effect on cancer cells and tumours as well as the application and granting of patents for the treatment of drug resistant cancer patients.[5]

That was what I had hoped to find because Cathy was a so-called drug resistant cancer patient as we knew by now.

Also, I came across some testimonials of patients from as far afield as Australia, Florida, USA, and Europe who stated that the ingestion of a minimal amount of 2.5mg of D,L-methadone had in the best case lead to a total apoptosis of their cancer, including brain cancer,[6] and in the worst case halted the growth and spread of multiple types of cancer.

---

[5] Use of opioids or opioid mimetics for the treatment of resistant cancer patients - US 8901175 B2
(*https://www.google.com/patents/US8901175*)

[6] Warum Methadon für Krebspatienten ein Hoffnungsschimmer ist
(*http://www.stern.de/tv/erfolge-in-der-tumorbehandlung--warum-methadon-fuer-manche-krebspatienten-ein-hoffnungsschimmer-ist-7501710.html*)

Out of sheer desperation I wrote a letter, a plea for help to Dr. Claudia Friesen, the researcher who had discovered the effect of D,L-methadone's properties so lethal to cancer. I was fully aware that her breakthrough results were achieved in the first instance with leukaemia but quite extensive retrospective and prospective trials with glioblastoma, the deadly brain cancer, and various other types of cancer, including oesophagus, kidney, and colorectal cancer, had been conducted with promising results. So, I hoped that these trials of the most difficult cancers to treat would include liver and bile duct cancer.

It took a few days for her to reply, which was no surprise when one considers that she was inundated with heartrending cries for help from around the world. What she wrote was a most considerate, detailed and very personal response, one would expect to receive from a friend.

She expressed her sorrow about Cathy's cancer, outlined the difficulties she faced, even from the German Cancer Society to have her research taken seriously as well as the positive results that had been achieved and were properly documented.

Funding for a complete and extensive clinical trial to provide proof of D,L-methadone's efficacy as an adjunct or adjuvant cancer drug had been denied at that time.

Various trials in Berlin, Munich, and Cologne had been done upon the initiative of the heads of university cancer clinics but did not include liver or bile duct cancer specifically.

She ended her message by informing me that doctors in Germany and neighbouring countries, I suppose she meant Poland, Czechia, Austria, Switzerland, France, Luxembourg, Belgium, Netherlands, and Denmark, were prescribing the aqueous solution of the medication for their cancer patients.

I investigated this last part of her message further and found that a vast number of doctors prescribed the medication for their cancer patients.

Our plan was now to stop over in Germany, visit a doctor near Frankfurt to have Cathy treated, and take some of the aqueous solution with us on our return to Canada.

But best-laid plans of mice and men often go awry... as the saying goes. That was certainly true in our case. First it was made abundantly clear that our tickets did not permit an extended layover and then I found out that methadone is a strictly controlled narcotic substance.

Should any methadone be found in our luggage upon our arrival in Canada, we would be arrested and thrown in prison for smuggling opioids despite a doctor's official prescription for cancer treatment.

Canadian customs officials were very keen on catching any drug smuggler in those days of 2016. Today, of course, Canadians just freak out when somebody lights up a cigarette or other tobacco product, while the smoking of marijuana "for recreation" and the ingestion of cannabis derivatives is actively promoted.

Crazy world, isn't it?

We concluded all our business in Riyadh on 15th October, our six suitcases were packed, and Sparky had been put into his carrier that was big enough for him and small enough to fit under the seat on the airplane in front of me. We loaded up the car and were ready to leave on our way to the international airport.

The guards of the housing compound gave us an emotional farewell with hugs and best wishes and many thanks for our household goods we had given them.

It was a drive in a melancholic mood past the lights of the shops and malls so familiar to us, along Khurais Road, the Eastern Ring Road, and the Airport Road.

While we waited at the check-in counter at the airport, my good friend Saud gave me a call. He apologised for not being able to make it in time with his entire family to see us off. I am sure he was crying unless he had developed a severe case of the sniffles.

Cathy's very good friend and colleague, Sa'ama called as well for a tearful farewell and to express her hope that we would be back soon.

We had made really good friends in this very intriguing and so often despised and condemned country. By our western standards not much is just dandy in Saudi Arabia but the people, by that I mean the regular Saudi citizens, are simply wonderful with very few exceptions.

Back in our Old Haunt

The flight and our entry into Canada behind us, we settled into a rented abode in the western rural area of the capitol region of Ottawa. Getting our stuff out of storage and making the place feel a bit like a real home took about a week.

Then we were off again to Toronto for another CT scan and an appointment with the radiologist and the surgeon. The scan had to be done to see if there had been any change in the status of the cancer.

We were told that a scrutiny of the scan pictures of some six weeks earlier had revealed in the radiologist's opinion that the diagnosis of bile duct cancer by Dr. Khaled and Dr. Mohammed could not be substantiated. Upon the question if the large tumour was inside or outside the liver, the answer was that it "appears" to be outside the liver but that could not be absolutely ascertained. Therefore, in their opinion it was safe to assume that it was liver cancer.

What? Safe to assume? What kind of pissy little screens do they have in that world-renowned cancer centre to view CT scan pictures? Don't they have a humongous screen that permits them to enlarge the pictures and see every detail in a three-dimensional format? It appeared that they don't have such advanced technology at their disposal, which is no surprise in view of the pretty well constant slashing of health care budgets in Canada.

On the other hand, the consultation with the surgeon turned out to be quite positive. He had reviewed the medical record and the CT scans and provided the optimistic outlook that Cathy could be a candidate for surgery of the liver and the spleen.

When he mentioned the spleen, I told him that at least three doctors in Riyadh had come to the conclusion that the growth was benign. He said that it was not what the medical record stated. Neither was there any mention of the possibility of bile duct cancer. That came as a surprise to us but at least the surgeon suggested a biopsy of the growth on the spleen to rule out any further misdiagnosis in that regard.

What a relief it was to have that specialist agree with me at least on that assertion. It was done the same afternoon and we were back on our way to Ottawa.

A few days later Cathy was informed that the growth on the spleen was indeed benign. That was a comfort because we expected that from that moment on the focus would be on a final investigation to determine if it was liver or bile duct cancer.

We couldn't have been more off base on that expectation. Bile duct cancer was never again taken into consideration by any of the doctors we consulted.

This procedure of going to Toronto for another consultation about every two weeks continued for the next five months. So, the seasonal music on the car radio changed from the usual fare of schmaltzy pop to the almost unbearable end-of-year muzak with some clown singing that winter is the best time of the year. It is doubtful he would vouch for the truth of his lyrics once he had to drive along Canada's busiest highway through the muck and blinding snow of a blizzard and make it on time to the next appointment with a surgeon.

There was no progress and we were given no indication when Cathy would be due for the surgery we still hoped could be performed. But everything we were told, which was essentially nothing new, during visit after visit became gloomier and gloomier.

The surgeon's station was overrun with patients all hoping for a miracle he could achieve only in the fewest of cases. I felt sorry for the doctor because he was totally overworked. He didn't like it when I mentioned that he looked overdue for a vacation. My inquiry if a treatment with medication for bile duct cancer wouldn't hold more promise to be effective or if at least the aqueous solution D,L-methadone could be prescribed, was dismissed with a look that told me to go back to the waiting room and count my fingers and toes. How dare you patronise a famous liver cancer surgeon?

I would come across that attitude and worse in the coming months of Cathy's slow but certain slide downhill.

Evidently the surgeon and his staff had fallen back on relying on the misdiagnosis of that doctor in the Hepatology Ward of the King Abdullah Hospital in Riyadh.

I don't want to be too hard on these specialists in Toronto. I suppose when one is utterly overworked and confronted by literally hundreds of cancer cases almost every day, it is very tempting to rely on the diagnosis of someone claiming to be a liver cancer specialist instead of proceeding with a lengthy and difficult investigation and arriving at one's own conclusions.

The worst outcome of these five months of regular visits was not getting any updates of Cathy's condition, no diagnosis, no prognosis. And nothing was done or even considered to slow the growth or cause the apoptosis of the cancer tumours. We, the patient and caregiver, were simply pushed along like a couple of items on a conveyor belt. It was just another complete waste of time.

We were told in March 2017 that surgery was out of the question and were handed a referral to the Cancer Ward of the Ottawa Hospital.

I still have great difficulty understanding the sole focus on liver cancer at the hospital in Toronto. During our first visit there after our return to Canada, the radiologist had stated that the large tumour appeared to be extrahepatic. Why wasn't that possibility investigated further? If it were outside the liver, then the diagnosis would have been bile duct cancer, not liver cancer. Should that have made a resection of the liver impossible, as many specialists state, then another surgeon should have been called upon to consider a bypass operation, whereby the surgeon connects a part of the bile duct, hepatic artery, or portal vein above the prime tumour with a part that is situated below the tumour. It would have had the benefit of cutting off the blood supply to the tumour, thus starving it, and possibly causing its apoptosis. Then the focus would have been only on the relatively small metastasis tumours that could quite possibly have been eradicated with cryosurgery or a NanoKnife.

These procedures I would have taken into consideration had I had any say in that matter. But then again, I am not a cancer surgeon or oncologist. Yet, it would have been reassuring had the focus of those specialists in Toronto not been solely and adamantly on a quack's misdiagnosis of liver cancer.

On Home Turf to the Bitter End

In preparation of our visits to the cancer centre in Ottawa, I printed out almost all the reports I had gathered in my global search for effective cancer treatments. Prominently featured were scientific reports of D,L-methadone, the successful palliative care treatment of over 5,000 cancer patients in a hospice in Germany[7] over a period of more than ten years as well as an analysis of the retrospective trial with glioblastoma patients[8] in Berlin's Charité Hospital. It made quite interesting reading for anyone bothering to study it but in the end hardly anybody appeared to have read it. It was all just foreign research and thus could be safely discarded as irrelevant.

The first visit to the cancer centre was not entirely disappointing. The oncologist was optimistic that not everything was lost. But despite a whole pile of CT scans on file, he insisted that another one had to be done.

What was the matter with these doctors? Didn't they trust each other's scans? I had lost count and it was anybody's guess of how many of the same pictures of Cathy's liver were now in her medical file. Still, we obliged and had to go to another hospital for the procedure.

During the following visits the oncologist was almost enthusiastic about a potential cure with one or another of the trial medications offered free of charge by Big Pharma. Had we known at that time of Prof. Zajicek's[9] advice to avoid participating in clinical trials, Cathy would not have become another guinea pig.

---

[7] Methadone: A misunderstood analgesic - with anti-tumor effects
  Gerda Kneifel, Medscape, 20th July 2017

[8] Safety and Tolerance of D,L-Methadone in Combination with Chemotherapy in Patients with Glioma, *Anticancer Research   March 2017 (https://www.reserachgate.net/publication/315204926)*

[9] Most new Oncology Drugs do not cure Cancer
  Gershom Zajicek, M.D., Professor of Experimental Medicine and Cancer Research, Faculty of Medicine, Hebrew University of Jerusalem

Prof. Zajicek states very bluntly that clinical trials are designed to use participants, not to help them. A clinical trial goes through the three phases of checking whether the drug works, checking its toxicity while ignoring, i.e. not recording and keeping track of the participants' suffering, and finally comparing the trial drug to other drugs that have been proven to work. He knows from experience that most of the tested new cancer drugs will not be approved, which means that the participants are subjected to a worthless trial that does more harm than good. He concludes that a clinical trial is an indicator of an oncologist betraying his mission of healing his patients.

It has to be made clear that Prof. Zajicek is not some know-all who wants to make a name for himself by mouthing off against Big Pharma. He is the professor of experimental medicine and cancer research at one of Israel's leading universities in this field.

Cathy went through all the trials. As could have been expected according to Zajicek's warning, they did not yield any positive results or the slightest improvement of her condition. Also, a review of her cancer file by a committee of doctors to consider a resection of her liver turned out to be negative, which was not surprising since the focus was again solely on liver cancer. The possibility of it being bile duct cancer was never taken into account.

The oncologist maintained his optimistic outlook and kept on searching for other trials that held any promise of slowing the growth or causing the apoptosis of the tumours. But fortunately for one or another reason it turned out that Cathy was not eligible for any of these trials because of the radio- and chemotherapy she had undergone.

So, he recommended an established medication that might be effective, and he wanted Cathy to give it a try. Having learned about the European Medicines Agency's review of medications to assess their efficacy or lack of it and its resoundingly negative outcome, I asked him what chance of success Cathy could expect with the recommended and very expensive medication that wasn't specifically for the treatment of liver or bile duct cancer but a so-called broad-spectrum drug.

He stated honestly that any cancer medication was only effective in about seventeen percent of cancer patient and provided a life extension of up to three and a half months on average.

We thanked him for his honesty, and I inquired about administering D,L-methadone. He responded to my query with a shrug, muttered something of it not being available in Canada, and we went home quite befuddled about what was to come next. And then things turned quite nasty. Cathy became weaker as time went by and the yellow discolouration returned to her face and eyes.

During our next consultation, the oncologist declared that draining the bile could not be done. He did not provide any reason for his decision or evidence of a diagnosis.

I handed him the pile of reports I had printed out and asked him again about the treatment with D,L-methadone because it had shown so much success in Germany. He appeared to take this suggestion as a personal affront and sharply asked quite peeved if we intended to go to Germany, flipped through the scientific reports without showing any interest and put them aside.

I assured him that a trip to Germany would be a last resort and that we were hoping to have the aqueous solution prescribed and administered in Canada. He stated that he could not prescribe that medication. It required a special license issued by the ministry of health that he did not have. Neither did he make a move to refer us to a colleague who had the license and could prescribe it upon his recommendation.

That was once more the end of the road at least with this oncologist who until that moment had been so encouraging and friendly. The bias against anything German, except cars, medical machinery, and bratwurst sits deep in Canada and became quite obvious with the oncologist.

As a follow-up we were confronted by a mealy-mouthing doctor talking to us about death and the inevitability of having to prepare for it.

I became quite outraged and asked if she meant that they had given up on treating Cathy and refused to explore every avenue still open. She should try to persuade a colleague or give us the name and address of a doctor in Canada who would prescribe D,L-methadone. Probably she had never heard of such medication and responded with a blank stare.

The peculiar development in this saga of a special license required for prescribing methadone was the declaration by the minister of health less than a year later that such a license was no longer needed. With a stroke of a pen she had repealed that law in response to her panic about the epidemic of some 4,000 opioid dependent Canadians killed with an overdose of Fentanyl in one year. There were two important facts she ignored or of which she was not aware. Firstly, while she gave her long public announcement of about an hour some 10 Canadians had died of cancer or one every six minutes, which adds up to 4,000 Canadians dying of that disease in just over two weeks and a total of over 83,000 that year. Secondly, she was ignorant of the difference of L-methadone, D-methadone, and D,L-methadone and the fact that only L-methadone is and should be used for the substitution therapy of opioid drug addicts.

What was the solution to our dilemma of not getting the treatment that had the potential of at least giving Cathy a life extension and an improvement of her quality of life? We were thinking about the last resort of going to Germany despite Cathy's deteriorating condition.

In preparation of such a move, I called Dr. Hilscher, the collaborator of Dr. Friesen with whom he had developed the aqueous solution he administered in appropriately safe dosages to the cancer patients in his hospice. I wanted to know if my wife could become his patient. Sadly, that was not possible. He explained that German law prohibits opioid treatment of non-resident foreigners who are not hospitalised in Germany or to prescribe opioids for them.

The doctor asked if I had presented the scientific reports of laboratory research, retrospective and prospective trial results to his Canadian peers, as well as his successful treatment of over 5,000 patients with D,L-methadone. I confirmed it and he asked why on the strength of the evidence of the reports they wouldn't prescribe the aqueous solution and administer it at the recommended dosage.

I replied that he was evidently not familiar with the arrogance or was it the inferiority complex of most Canadian doctors who view essentially any medical research done and results achieved outside of Canada and especially in Germany as piffle unless it comes from Big Pharma. They all appear to live in their own little ice block igloo solidly frozen shut to any outside influence.

He laughed at my poor joke and suggested to go to the States where most doctors would prescribe it instantly. I explained that I would then have to bring the supply of aqueous solution methadone into Canada, which would land me for several years in prison for smuggling narcotics.

After his encouraging words not to give up my search for a Canadian doctor willing to prescribe the medication because there must be someone who would oblige we ended our cordial conversation.

Adhering to his advice I began a search for doctors and clinics that could possibly prescribe the desired medication. But every inquiry was answered in the negative.

Palliative Care - The Second

The next visit to the cancer centre brought us an unexpected turn of events. The oncologist had ended the consultations without informing us beforehand about his decision. It furthered my suspicion that he had not been entirely open and honest with us about Cathy's condition.

Instead of the oncologist we met a palliative care specialist. That was a really bad development.

During the consultation with the palliative care doctor I asked him right off the bat if he was licensed to prescribe D,L-methadone. He confirmed to be licensed and gave me a very suspicious look. I told him about the treatment in Germany and that we wanted to try it for Cathy as a last resort. He waved it off and said that the required hydrochloride powder was not available in Canada.

I did not believe him and mentioned that my research included a report from the province of Alberta that showed that every type of methadone was available in Canada. I would provide him the entire lot of scientific reports I had gathered.

He expressed no interest but gave us a long lecture about the palliative care I would have to provide in our home environment. Then he left and sent in his assistant, an intern on the cusp of becoming another palliative care specialist.

We were not impressed by her performance. First she wanted to prescribe the broad-spectrum anti-cancer medication that had already been established as useless and would cost us several thousand bucks a shot. Then she insisted on prescribing morphine for Cathy's pain management although Cathy expressed firmly that she did not suffer any pain but was very concerned about the quite evidently rising bilirubin count.

When Cathy asked for a prescription of bilirubin binding medication, the intern looked as if she had never heard of such a thing. Then I told her if she was busy prescribing the medicine requested by Cathy, she should add the aqueous

64

solution D,L-methadone and showed her Dr. Hilscher's detailed prescription. The up-and-coming palliative care specialist stared at the paper that she only needed to sign and stamp to turn it into a valid prescription until she was asked to reveal which pharmacy would have the hydrochloride powder and could prepare the racemic aqueous solution.

With a look of a sourpuss upset about being confronted by a couple that was knowledgeable about cancer and bilirubin she said, "No way! We stick to the tried and true!"

With 'we' she presumably referred to her boss and herself unless in a hint of megalomania she referred to the entire medical profession of Canada.

She tore her morphine prescription off the block, thrust it into Cathy's hand, and walked out without another word.

We didn't know if anyone wanted to talk to us after this encounter of the weird kind, waited for about ten minutes, and then left as well. Cathy assured me that she was never going to take morphine or even bother to get it.

Upon our return home I packed the whole pile of methadone information into an envelope, scribbled the palliative care specialist's name and the message "Read it, please. It is very urgent!" on it, rushed back to the hospital and dropped it off in his office. I don't know if he ever read any of the reports since I never got a response from him.

A couple of days later another palliative care specialist phoned us to announce that she was in charge of the care for Cathy and inquired about her condition. I explained that she needed either draining her bilirubin or bile binding medication as well as D,L-methadone.

She ignored the request for the medicines but stated that she wanted to meet us for a detailed discussion. A date was arranged for a meeting two days later.

Another phone call from the Ottawa Hospital informed us that we didn't need to show up at the palliative care ward any longer. Instead we were supposed to see a general practitioner in the hospital of the small town of Arnprior, west of our place of residence. An appointment for the next day had already been arranged. So, we went to see the doctor. In preparation of the visit, I took along another pile of the methadone research reports for him.

He was friendly enough and wanted Cathy to tell him what she had planned for the future. That was a strange request since he didn't specify what future he had in mind. Did he know of a miraculous cure and referred to years of her life after she was healed, or did he refer to the next three days and expected her to collapse any minute? We should find out just a few days later that it had been merely polite conversation to make Cathy feel at ease.

When I raised the topic of methadone, he didn't wave it off and even pretended to know about it. But in short order I found out that he only knew about the drug addiction substitute and had no idea that there were three types of methadone with distinctly different applications. I handed him the envelope full of reports and he promised to read all of it while he stated that he didn't have the license to prescribe the aqueous solution and doubted that the hydrochloride powder was available in Canada.

The next day we met the doctor in charge of Cathy's palliative care. A lengthy woman-to-woman conversation between her and my wife took place that would have been beyond the comprehension of most people, I presume, because no specific point of an envisaged treatment was addressed.

Getting a bit fidgety about this endless talk and as soon as she mentioned morphine, I intervened asking her if she was licensed to prescribe methadone. Of course, she was. She enlightened us that palliative care specialists in Canada are the only medics licensed to prescribe that analgesic.

Encouraged I asked her if she had heard of or knew about D,L-methadone being used as an adjunct or adjuvant cancer medication. She did not need to answer. Her baffled look said that she had never heard of it.

I gave her the pile of reports, which sounds by now as if I had given all the doctors we had met the piles, which I hope I did as a reminder that there is an adjunct that alleviates the symptoms of cancer and potentially provides a cure. I asked her to read the entire volume of scientific reports and prescribe the aqueous solution D,L-methadone, the only medication holding the promise of helping Cathy.

For a second I thought a fire alarm had gone off before she went into a mad rant about the life-threatening dangers of administering methadone. When she explained that as little as 40mg could kill Cathy instantly, I stopped her to ask if she knew the difference between the different types of methadone. She insisted that it was all the same. So, there I was, a medical layman, having to explain to a Canadian palliative care specialist with years of experience of administering the deadly opioids morphine and fentanyl the difference of L-methadone as a substitution for opioid dependants, D-methadone for nerve disorders, and D,L-methadone and its application for cancer. I am certain that she didn't hear a word I said.

She insisted that a methadone treatment of 10mg a day had to be administered by a highly trained nurse once a day, thus implying that it had to be administered intravenously, which was not possible due to the shortage of staff.

I corrected her assertion by referring to the report of an investigation of Canadian cancer specialists of some 18 years earlier[10] wherein they concluded that methadone was safe for outpatient titration without specifying the need of intravenous drug administration once a day by a trained nurse.

---

[10] Methadone: Outpatient Titration and Monitoring Strategies in Cancer Patients, *5th November 1999*
Neil A. Hagen, MD, FRCPC, and Eric Wasylenko, MD, Division of Palliative Medicine, Department of Oncology, University of Calgary, Alberta, Journal of Pain and Symptom Management

Moreover, I explained that the aqueous solution D,L-methadone had to be administered sublingually and would start in Cathy's case with 2.5mg twice a day, i.e. every twelve hours, together with ten percent of the recommended dosage of her anti-cancer medication. The quantity of methadone should be raised over several days to a maximum of 20mg per day according to Cathy's response and only if she took to it well. So, 40mg a day was completely out of the question.

That good doctor was by now royally pissed off with me. Here was a guy without medical training providing more specifics about a medication and administering it properly as a cancer adjunct then she had ever known in her entire miserable life as a highly touted palliative care specialist. She gave Cathy a prescription for morphine to help her sleep, said that she would be in touch, and left.

The following day I went to the local pharmacy to pick up the sedative. Instead of the diluted morphine, the pharmacist had received a tiny bottle of highly concentrated morphine. She suggested that I should be very careful with it and give my wife only a drop or two. I gave the bottle back because I had no intention of following her advice. The slightest slip-up would have killed Cathy and landed me in prison on a murder charge.

I presented the recipe for the aqueous solution and explained to the pharmacist that it had to be made with 1g of hydrochloride powder D,L-methadone dissolved in 100ml purified water with minute amounts of ascorbic and citric acid and put into a pipette bottle for the control of drops. The pharmacist confirmed that she could prepare it upon presentation of a prescription but said that the hydrochloride powder was not available in Canada to the best of her knowledge.

While I was in the pharmacy, the doctor called to tell me about a new anti-cancer drug one of the Big Pharma companies claimed to have developed. I said that we were not interested in any of these allegedly new wonder drugs at outrageous prices. We had no intention to waste our money on such stuff.

I pleaded with her to consider the methadone recipe that was now in her possession and let us have a prescription as quickly as possible. She finally relented and promised to have a prescription and the methadone sent to the pharmacy the next day, a Saturday. A special delivery arrived late at night with hundreds of syringes for administering the exact amount of the aqueous solution sublingually because they didn't have any pipette bottles.

Full of hope to have reached the apex of our struggle I went to the pharmacy on Saturday. The pharmacist wasn't in. The young assistant in her place assured me that she had received the medicine but was not allowed to prepare the solution.

Because I had never seen the hydrochloride powder, I asked her to show me what had been delivered. She obliged and came back with a big bottle labelled 'Methadol'. I was stunned and couldn't believe it. To make sure that she hadn't made a mistake, I asked her if a pouch or small container of hydrochloride powder had not been delivered?

No, that bottle was everything she had received and confirmed that the pharmacist intended to use that liquid for the preparation of the aqueous solution. That was beyond me and I told her that the recipe I had left with the pharmacy could only be prepared with hydrochloride powder. The liquid in that bottle is used in its full strength as an opioid substitute for drug addicts. I asked her how many millilitres of methadol would be the exact equivalent of 1g of hydrochloride powder. She did not know. According to my swift calculation a quantity of between 20ml and 100ml of methadol could be equivalent to 1g of powder since the exact strength of the liquid was not specified. Mixing it with 100ml of purified water would result in a deviation from the prescribed recipe, the proven result of more than ten years of research and given with great success to over 5,000 cancer patients. It would prove to be useless, if it was too weak, or could kill my wife instantly, if it was too strong. I was unwilling to take that risk.

Desperately I tried to phone the palliative care specialist to let her know about the mistake. Every number I dialled was answered by a machine informing me about the office hours from Monday to Friday. That was all I needed to have my suspicions confirmed that a quiet weekend was more important to that palliative care specialist than caring for a seriously ill patient.

Cathy's condition had worsened. She was now shaken by being ice cold one moment and suffering sudden heat flashes the next with a high temperature of over 40° Celsius lasting more than an hour.

Despite her massive problems she had managed to complete the forms for having her remains donated to science and her last will and testament. The forms had to be witnessed and the following Monday, 27th November, we went to see the doctor in Arnprior. He and a nurse obliged to sign the papers as witnesses.

The doctor was quite shocked to notice Cathy's deteriorating condition but couldn't do anything about it. I told him about the methadol delivery instead of methadone hydrochloride powder and asked him to call the palliative care specialist because I could not reach her by phone even during her office hours. He tried to defend his medical colleague by repeating her claim that the hydrochloride powder was not available in Canada.

Undeterred by all the setbacks I continued my search for the methadone we wanted. I went as far as calling manufacturers in Switzerland, France, Scotland, Cuba, and the United States. All the manufacturers that could supply it understood my problem but explained that a shipment of less than 10kg would not be considered and that any order had to be placed by the national health authority.

Cathy's friend Alison had been visiting us. Her sister was a nurse and had all sorts of contacts in and knowledge of the medical drug supply system. She promised to look into it and send whatever information she could find.

Valuable time was ticking away, and I didn't make any progress the next few days. On Thursday, 30th November, I received a call from the doctor in Arnprior inquiring if we had considered delivering Cathy to a hospice. No, we had not, and I discussed his suggestion with my wife.

It was all up in the air until Cathy said, "I don't want to die in this house."

That statement hit me square in the face. Cathy had given up on ever getting better or healed.

The doctor called again in the morning of Friday, 1st December, and told us that there was a vacancy in a hospice that was so good that he would want to be submitted there himself whenever it should become necessary. Putting that gobbledegook aside, I asked him if a doctor could and would administer D,L-methadone there.

Almost enthusiastically he assured me that the doctor in charge at the hospice was licensed, familiar with the medication, and would definitely administer it. That clinched it. Assured that Cathy would at last be given a curative therapy and treatment, we agreed to have her submitted to the hospice.

Little did we know...

The Final Days

An ambulance was not required. I let our car warm up to assure Cathy's comfort, sat her down, and we went on a very solemn 30km drive to the hospice. Once I had found the proper entrance to the low building, a nurse brought out a wheelchair, sat Cathy down, and pushed her inside. While she was brought to her room and helped to go to bed, I filled in the forms to the satisfaction of the little old lady at the reception and handed her all the documentation required.

Cathy's room was bright and spacious, and she looked almost content tucked into a comfortable single bed. It looked very promising to be the right place for her care although I was a bit surprised about the absence of any equipment one would normally see in a hospital room. No monitors, no warning systems, nothing. Still, we had a lovely chat full of optimism that everything would turn out all right now. She reminded me to look after Sparky, our cat, really well. He was for now, as she emphasised, my only companion.

And then the doctor that was assigned to look after her made an appearance. Dressed entirely in black and with her long black hair dangling about, she looked like a malevolent Dr. Death. She did not inspire any confidence.

Ignoring me and without introducing herself, she pulled up a chair next to the bedside, and told Cathy to stretch out her left arm and push up the sleeve. She prepared a syringe and looked for a vein. Before she injected the medication, I asked her what that was. I had to ask her twice before she bothered to look at me askance like a bothersome insect and said, "Fentanyl."

Very firmly I told her to stop that immediately. Cathy was to be treated with the aqueous solution D,L-methadone that had to be administered sublingually. We had been promised by her colleague in Arnprior that she, the doctor would know about that drug, have it, and administer it. Fentanyl was proven to be a totally useless analgesic unless one wants to commit suicide with an overdose, and it was contraindicative for the treatment of cancer.

She actually bothered to turn around and face me properly to tell me that I had no say in this matter and neither did a general practitioner had any say in the treatment of her patients in the hospice. As an experienced palliative care specialist who had interned and practised in Alberta she knew best what was right, she said and claimed that methadone was not available in Canada or suitable for cancer treatment.

I wondered then and still do so if Dr. Death had ever taken the 'Hippocratic Oath'[11] or sworn to abide by the 'Code of Medical Ethics'[12], which states in Section 8, "A physician should seek consultation upon request in doubtful or difficult cases or whenever it appears that the quality of medical service may be enhanced thereby." And the GP in Arnprior should have observed Section 4 of the code that states, "The medical professional should safeguard the public and itself against physicians deficient in moral character or professional competence."

Dr. Death poked the needle into Cathy's arm, pumped the Fentanyl in, and left. Within minutes Cathy was in what I can only describe as a drug induced coma.

Outraged I went to see the head nurse and wanted to know who the boss was, the superior of this alleged doctor. She couldn't or didn't want to tell me but assured me that Cathy was in the best of care.

That was a load of bullshit as I could see when I went back to see my wife. She did not respond when I talked to her. In the hope that she would at least have a good rest and be better in the morning, I left to go home.

---

[11] Hippocratic Oath
   (https://www.britannica.com/topic/Hippocratic-oath)
[12] The Code of Medical Ethics of the American Medical Association
   (https://www.ncbi.nlm.nih.gov/pmc/articles/PMC3399321/)

Over the weekend it appeared that Cathy's condition was improving. She sat up in bed and we had a pleasant conversation although I noticed that she slurred her words. She wanted better food and said that she missed the meals I had always prepared for her.

I told her about my continued search for a source that could supply methadone and assured her that once I found it, she would be treated with it and soon get better.

Sunday night she asked me to brush her hair, which I did cautiously and with great care. Before I left, I told her that I loved her, and she confirmed that she loved me too.

Those were the last words we exchanged face to face.

On Monday, 4th December 2017, early in the morning Cathy called me. I was pleasantly surprised how crisp and clear her voice sounded when she asked me to bring her some pudding they didn't have in the hospice. Yes, of course, I would do that. I had to check the e-mail responses to my inquiries quickly and would see her in a little while.

That's when I heard her scream to someone, "What the hell are you doing?" The call was abruptly ended, and her phone was shut down. Several times I tried to reach the hospice by phone, but nobody answered as if they knew what was in store for them.

Among the e-mails was the helpful message from Cathy's friend Alison with several telephone numbers in Ottawa of people who might know where to get methadone.

I called the first number and noticed that the woman answering was very reluctant to talk to me. Later I found out it was a safe house for domestically abused women. I briefly explained that I called in the hope that she could help me with some information about obtaining D,L-methadone for my wife who was in a hospice stricken with cancer.

Her tone changed to almost warm and she gave me the telephone number of people who could help me. My next call was answered by a woman who assured me that a select number of pharmacies with a clientele of people addicted to opioids would have the medicine I wanted. She gave me three numbers to call.

Before I could contact one of these pharmacies, the hospice called to let me know that my wife had taken a turn for the worse. I wanted to know what had happened and tell her that I would be on my way almost instantly. My question was not answered, and the call was cut short.

Feeling under extreme pressure, I called the first pharmacy, rattled off the prescription for the aqueous solution, and asked if they could help me.

Of course, confirmed the pharmacist, they had the hydrochloride powder in stock and could deliver the aqueous solution in a pipette bottle within an hour upon presentation of a doctor's prescription.

YES!! YES!!! I had finally found the source of the medication I had tried to find for over a year. It was thanks to an underground network of people willing to help each other.

It provided proof that all those medics who had stated that the hydrochloride powder was not available in Canada had either been totally ignorant or a bunch of rotten liars with ulterior motives and extreme bias. Now I could go to confront Dr. Death with the news and demand that she write the required prescription.

I was ready to rush to Cathy's side with the good news and on the doorstep, when the telephone rang. It was a hospice nurse who informed me curtly that my wife had passed away and hung up.

I was completely devastated. The light of my life had been extinguished.

I don't remember how I drove the 30km to the hospice without getting involved in an accident. But I do remember the moment I walked into the room and saw Cathy.

I burst into tears and my uncontrolled grief and pain gave a nurse sufficient cause to shut the door with a bang. The hospice staff was evidently not used to or uncomfortable with such undignified outburst of emotions.

In the afternoon there was a meeting with the nurses and Dr. Death. I berated that quack with quite a few choice insults and finally barged into her with the question if she was happy now that she had so quickly dispatched another one of her patients with a useless drug in less than four days. Nobody said a word. All the nurses just stared at me and not one was answering my questions of who had shut down Cathy's phone after she had screamed her last question and why she had screamed. Dr. Death was utterly unperturbed and checked her shoes with a sardonic smile on her face.

Late in the evening a funeral home took care of Cathy's remains and shipped it to the Department of Anatomy of the University of Ottawa according to the instructions Cathy had written a week before her death.

I was glad to get out of that house of horrors at last. I went to our abode that did not feel like a home any longer. Sparky seemed to sense my pain, cuddled up to me, and purred. Was he trying to sooth my soul? I don't know but I was glad to have him as a companion in my darkest hour.

Aftermath

There is not much more to be said about Cathy's case history of cancer treatment gone horribly wrong except that it provides a glimpse of Canada's much touted and lauded universal health care system.

The statement of a doctor[13] who practises in Canada's northern Ontario provides a confirmation of my criticism. "The system isn't broken, the system is doing what it was originally designed to do," says Dr. Mike Kirlew. "It was never meant to provide care. It was meant to deny care. They have this phrase in medicine called the Hippocratic Oath. We take it when we graduate from medical school. It means 'to do no harm'. Sometimes I see my role as a physician to minimize the harm that the system is already doing to [the patients]."

That applies to Dr. Kirlew's patients and certainly applied to Cathy as well. I wish that some of the American and Canadian promoters of the health care system would pay more attention to the lack of critical care and not only to the aspect of money. Of course, it is nice and exemplary not to be presented with a multi-million-dollar bill after doctors failed miserably at their job. But with the conservative element of Canada's society and various conservative governments constantly demanding a reduction in taxes and, as a first measure in this endeavour, the slashing of health care budgets, it is little wonder that the health insurance program is by no means what it could or should be.

This is confirmed by many reports about treatment of a range of medical problems and diseases gone wrong. These reports are not presented by a press antagonistic to universal health care. On the contrary, they are produced by journalists that would in all likelihood fight in the trenches to defend

---

[13] Health system neglects northern patients by design: Doctor *Nick Purdon & Leonardo Palleja, CBC News, 10th March 2018 (https://www.cbc.ca/news/canada/north/north-health-care-system-problems-1.4523140)*

Canada's health care system. But they point out the problems and shortcomings of the health insurance program and suggest that it should be improved with a massive financing increase and much less bureaucracy.

The major failure in Ontario's health-care system was addressed with a report[14] about a cancer patient who had to seek treatment in the USA. It underscores the problem of the breakdown of an essential cancer care program in Ontario hospitals due to the lack of sufficient financing. Since the early 1990s, doctors had repeatedly warned the health ministry about this inevitable collision between inadequate resources and "unprecedented demand", but the crisis went largely unaddressed. They pleaded for extra government funds through internal memos and reports for more than a decade to perform allogeneic transplants on patients, which use stem cells for cancer treatment from unrelated donors. Cancer Care Ontario, the government agency responsible for overseeing this program, would not say how many of the patients that had been approved for out-of-country treatment had relapsed due to excessive bureaucratic procedures before being admitted to a hospital in the USA and thus could not be treated with the stem cell transplant required for their specific type of cancer. The agency's spokeswoman claimed to be unable to provide this number due to patient privacy.

Also, that Cathy's case is not an exceptional event undeserving of any attention is the first-hand account of a cancer patient[15], who I hope is still alive and recovering. It bears an uncanny resemblance to Cathy's case history. In

---

[14] Sharon's story: Trip to Buffalo for stem-cell transplant came too late *Toronto Star, Diana Zlomislic, 27ᵗʰ April 2016* *(https://www.thestar.com/news/gta/2016/04/27/sharons-story-trip-to-buffalo-for-stem-cell-transplant-came-too-late.html)*

[15] 'I chose to fight': She's doing all she can to find a cure for her ovarian cancer, *Tawsha Klein-Sparks, 26ᵗʰ Feb. 2020* *(https://www.cbc.ca/news/canada/edmonton/ cancer-tawsha-klein-sparks-edmonton-1.5463127)*

reference to the survival rate for her specific type of cancer that has not improved in over fifty years, the woman states, "This is an unacceptable statistic that needs to change."

I agree and don't need to add anything to her statement because it holds true for most types of cancer.

A few weeks after Cathy's death I contacted the hospice board with a request for my wife's entire medical record. I suspected foul play. Looking at the record my suspicions have never been entirely eliminated. The hand-scribbled entries with a pencil about how much or how little Fentanyl was pumped into Cathy did not convince me that they were the original entries or that every care had been taken to aim for a prolongation of her life. On the contrary!

Also, the notes of an interview that was conducted while Cathy was in a drug induced coma showed clearly that the interviewer imposed her own pathetic standards of religious beliefs and living the good life. It was a collection of falsehoods and insinuations that at first glance cast a despicably negative light on Cathy, but in reality, it just mirrored the pitiful life of the interviewer.

I wrote a summary of the false assessments, Dr. Death's shoddy, slapdash treatment, and highlighted in particular the lies and denials that had been presented to us by medical staff. I gave this summary to the director of the hospice board but never got a satisfactory answer or an apology during a meeting or in writing ever since.

Nothing less should have been expected. Not once were any of the doctors in charge entirely open with us about Cathy's deteriorating state of health. It made me think of the time some twenty years earlier in Germany when my mother was stricken with cancer. Every doctor involved in caring for her gave me complete assessments of the procedures, the likelihood of the outcome of applied therapies, and the advance of her illness. Never was I left in the dark about the chances of her survival. And when it was established that nothing could be done for her any longer, the oncologist in charge told me so in confidence. We had a long conversation, during which he explained that her cancer had metastasised out of control, that neither therapy nor medication that was available at that time could stop the spread and growth, and that she would die probably within two weeks.

My mother had signed a request to die in dignity in her home, a form letter equivalent to 'do not resuscitate' in other countries. I abided by her wishes, took her out of the hospital, and had her brought back to her abode by ambulance. I took care of her with the help of a professional care giver of the Red Cross, made the meals she enjoyed so much, had conversations with her that made her laugh, and as the oncologist had predicted she died peacefully in her sleep two weeks later. I appreciated the doctor having trusted me to have the strength to deal with the truth, told him so, and thanked him.

I would have been equally thankful to the doctors in charge of treating Cathy had they had the courage to be as open and supportive as their German counterpart had been so many years earlier. But honesty in the doctor-patient relationship is a matter of ongoing debate in North America although it is known that not telling the truth causes patients serious harm.

An example of that lack of support is a report[16] about a woman who died suddenly after four years of having been treated for breast cancer. Her husband summed up their horrendous experience with the words, "What she needed, and we needed was a deep conversation about what to expect." That did not happen. Instead, when he met with a palliative physician, he was told that feeding his wife would only feed her cancer. The next day he returned to the hospital to find that

---

[16] 'A terrible shock'
CBC Radio's Ottawa Morning, CBC News, 9th July 2017
(https://www.cbc.ca/news/canada/ottawa/palliative-care-paul-adams-ottawa-1.4191049)

his wife was no longer being hydrated, either. Not a word was lost that his wife had only a few days to live.

He stated that more work needs to be done to inform caregiver and patient about what to expect at the end of the patient's life and said, "You have to understand, when you're caring for somebody with cancer, you've devoted years of your life to nurturing them ... and [my wife's death] came as just a terrible, terrible shock.... I think that if I had been prepared for that it would have made a difference."

It is no consolation to find out belatedly that I am not the only caregiver who was kept totally in the dark about my wife's actual status and what to expect.

The phrase "We *can* no longer do anything for you", that was suggested to tell a patient, may have been appropriate many years ago. It is not applicable any longer. When all avenues of a potential cure with adjunct medications that could help alleviate suffering and have the potential of a curative effect are fiercely rejected, the phrase in all honesty should be, "We *will* no longer do anything for you."

As a consequence of the lack of honesty, patients lose that important trust which is required for healing. Honesty matters to patients. Most cancer patients in North America never receive information from their physicians about prognosis or imminent death. That lack of knowledge is associated with worse quality of care and worse quality of life for the patient and surviving caregivers.[17] It is also the significant difference of care between North America and Europe.

***

---

[17] Giving Honest Information to Patients with Advanced Cancer Maintains Hope
Thomas J. Smith, MD, Lindsay A. Dow, MD, James Khatcheressian, MD, Laurel J. Lyckholm, MD, Robin Matsuyama, PhD, 15th May 2010 (https://www.cancernetwork.com/end-life-care/giving-honest-information-patients-advanced-cancer-maintains-hope)

A final word as regards Cathy's Case History is necessary to balance the picture that was presented. It could create the impression that the health care systems of Canada as well as Saudi Arabia are dominated by uncaring, almost heartless professionals. Such pompous, callous, and self-centred professionals do exist, but they are not a majority.

In both countries and in every one of the other fifteen countries where I had the good fortune to work and live, the majority of medical practitioners are very caring, competent and dedicated professionals. I think in particular of Dr. Kirlew and doctors like him who practice in outlying areas under the most difficult of circumstances of any given country. They don't shy away from going to extreme length to care singlehandedly for three, four, or more communities and provide the best service their respective health care systems permit. This is particularly true for the frozen north, barren deserts, and similarly inhospitable regions of many other countries.

I have the greatest respect for these true professionals and salute every one of them as well as all those medical professionals who showed us some humility and true care in the execution of their duties.

Current Cancer Treatment and its Repercussions

It took some months for me to regain my composure and equilibrium after the harrowing experience of being unable to help my wife get healed and healthy again and seeing her wilt away. Her image of a woman, quiet and unassuming, stays with me practically every day. She had achieved so much more, academically with her master's degree and otherwise with her filmmaking and travels to exotic countries, than any member of her family, living or dead.

As far as the medics were concerned, I began to have the visual perception of most of them being one-eyed ogres who lacked any depth of vision and clung like obsessed to the misdiagnosis of a quack. It took a while to regain a balance of vision and see these people as humans incapable of jumping over their own shadow just like myself or anybody else.

I continued my research of cancer therapies conducted around the world. When I read some reports about successful treatments that are usually not very much publicised, I became determined to find out why the treatment of Cathy had failed so badly. At first I encountered a lot of very negative information that made me dream of a miraculous cure that sets everything right.

Suspend disbelief for a moment and imagine with me, if you will, after you were diagnosed with cancer and the review of the main tumour's DNA sequencing has been done by the oncologist, you receive the cheerful message that it is nothing to worry about.

Your cancer, no matter what type, will be eradicated and you will be healed within a few weeks at a cost of about $200 for an immune system therapy that has no side effects.

That is, of course, just a wonderful dream scenario. But will it or can it happen some day in the foreseeable future that we will have such a miraculous therapy?

Humanity can only hope that the researchers and doctors who are working tirelessly towards the goal of an effective and all-encompassing immunotherapy will develop a treatment still considered unattainable today. Once achieved, it would bring relief to the millions of people that are diagnosed with cancer every year and the many more millions that barely survive and are living with cancer.

While research is going on globally to find the panacea, the treatment of all types of cancer, it is in all likelihood a long way to go before a great and ultimate breakthrough will be discovered.

Cancer is a very complicated disease. It is not a one-off affliction that is the same for every human being and every part of the anatomy in contrast to some diseases that can be treated with one medication for all.

Current cancer research shows clearly that many aspects of cancer are only partially understood. It has been compared to a 100,000-piece jigsaw puzzle of which barely 1% of the pieces have been recognised and placed correctly.

Researchers and oncologists agree that cancer is a corrupted version of healthy cells, mutations of DNA that change until the cells grow, divide uncontrollably, and endanger health and life of the patient. But the verdict is still out why healthy cells suddenly become cancerous. The uncontrolled growth and the rapid spread of cancer cells also still pose many questions.

A ten-year global study titled "Pan-Cancer Analysis of Whole Genomes"[18] was conducted by a consortium of more than a thousand scientists carrying out their research at over

---

[18] Pan-cancer analysis of whole genomes, *5th Feb 2020*
    (https://www.nature.com/articles/s41586-020-1969-6)

seven hundred institutions. The result was published in February 2020. It concluded that cancer is massively complex with thousands of different combinations of mutations able to cause cancer tumours.

The scientists found some fundamental mutations that drive a cancer's growth and could be exploited to identify treatments that are tailored to each individual patient.

Carbon dating these fundamental mutations showed that about 20% of them occur decades before a cancer tumour is recognised. It is now a matter of identifying, which one of these mutations become cancer tumours and which ones can be safely ignored to avoid overdiagnosis and the treatment of patients whose innate immune system is fully capable of dealing with and destroying cancer cells.

The study has shown the path of the work ahead to achieve the ultimate breakthrough that will heal patients of their cancer. It is a long and winding path that will take many years to be covered.

At present, with more than 200 identified types of cancer, whose cause is mostly unknown, what is done mainly is the removal of large tumours with invasive surgery, destroy small cancer cells with cryosurgery[19] or the NanoKnife[20], apply various highly toxic chemotherapies and radiotherapy in the hope of preventing the spread and growth of cancer and killing cancer cells. This treatment of cancer appears to be straightforward and simple. Yet it has been proven to be delusional since millions of cancer patients die every year after having been "effectively" treated with such conventional cancer therapies.

---

[19] Cryosurgery is a type of surgery that involves the use of extreme cold to destroy abnormal tissues, such as tumours, *8th July 2017 (www.healthline.com/health/cryosurgery)*

[20] The NanoKnife System is an ablative device that uses IRE (Irreversible Electroporation) technology to achieve cell death. *(nanoknife.com)*

No Cure for Cancer - Yet

Two hundred types of cancer identified to date could lead one to surmise that there are about two hundred different types of cancer cells. But there are many more because in every tumour there are millions of cells that mutate boundlessly and are very different from the cells of another tumour. And once these cancer cells spread to other sites in the body and settle on another organ or a different spot on the same organ, they develop into tumours with a unique structure of cells and their very own defence mechanisms.

Suddenly confronted with the devastating diagnosis of cancer, most people are despondent and feel panic, be it the person diagnosed, a family member, or the caregiver. In realisation of knowing very little, if anything about the disease, the fear sets in that nothing can be done to save the life of the patient - that this is the end! The fear is corroborated by almost daily media reports about failed treatments, the recurrence of cancer that had been "beaten"[21], as was the case of an entertainer in Australia who died, or the painful struggle of the quartet of an Irish family pop group in England[22] dealing with recurring cancer. The ultimate death of yet another famous person having succumbed to cancer is reported like a national tragedy while the other over 25,000 people who die from cancer around the world every day are listed as a statistic.

As soon as a cancer patient becomes aware of the relative hopelessness to be healed and that the cost of most oncologist recommended and prescribed medications will result in abject poverty, desperation takes over and the search for so-called "alternative" treatments and medications begins. And that is the first big mistake.

---

[21] The Australian entertainer Natasha Stuart dies aged 43
Sydney Morning Herald, 29ᵗʰ Jan. 2020
[22] Nolan sisters Linda and Anne undergoing cancer treatment
BBC News, 3ʳᵈ Aug. 2020

Firstly, these alternative treatments such as homeopathy, naturopathy, or anthropopathy ranging from ingesting diluted doses of substances that in larger amounts would produce symptoms of the ailment, pumping lemon juice into the veins, smoking pot until your eyeballs pop out, or intense prayer sessions under the guidance of some money grabbing guru or preacher are in their sum not any cheaper than Big Pharma medications. Secondly, none of them have ever undergone clinical trials or provided any proof of efficacy whatsoever.

It is remotely possible that one or another "natural substance" praised as the one and only to eradicate cancer may help to improve the patient's immune system. But again that has never been proven in empirical clinical trials.

So, my advice is simply to stay away from charlatans' wonder recipes and Aunt Hulda's advice to drink gallons of dandy lion root tea that she claims will simply wash away the tumours. It will do more damage to health and bank account then the conventional treatment that provides the slim sliver of hope of a short life extension.

Yet, the conventional cancer treatment of surgery (cut), radiation (burn), and chemotherapy (poison) does not provide a cure either in the sense of eradicating the cancer for good and restoring the patient's health.

Cut, burn, and poison is limited to removing the visible tumours, but it does not eradicate the cancer, specifically not the small cancer cells that have not been recognised as such and cannot be seen in the pictures of a CT scan.

You have to remember that every human being has at any time millions, even billions of cancer cells floating around in the body that are normally detected and eradicated by a healthy immune system. These tiny cancer cells escape eradication when the immune system is very weak or malfunctions.

Consequently, it is no surprise that cancer recurs, yet in more vicious forms because the cancer cells that survived the initial burning and poisoning of visible tumours have become immune to that treatment. Cancer cells develop many mechanisms to become resistant to drugs and radiation. They strengthen their defence system against any form of attack from chemotherapy and, far worse, the patient's immune system.

Therefore, it is preposterous to think and downright ludicrous to claim that a patient's cancer can be eradicated with surgery, radio- and chemotherapy, i.e. with cut, burn, and poison.

Surgery of a tumour or tumours is a very delicate, complicated, and costly operation. Only what has been clearly identified and is visible as a tumour as a result of a CT scan, be it a cancer tumour on its own or a number of tumours on an organ or part of an organ, can be removed by a surgeon.

That does not mean or even imply that the cancer has been eradicated because the success of surgery is limited by the mechanisms of the cancer spreading.

So, what about the remaining cancer cells that often are detected only after surgery?

Well, they are blasted with radiation in an attempt to kill them. But again, they are only those tumours that have become visible as a result of screening the patient and have been identified with a biopsy as cancerous. And however carefully the radiotherapy is conducted it has a detrimental effect on healthy tissue.

Also, the billions of cancer cells that are at an early stage of development and a result of the incessant division of cancer cells are not affected. They can't be detected or made visible with today's medical technology.

So, what about these nasty little 'terrorists' in waiting?

Ah-hah, here comes Big Pharma's chemotherapy, the poison trusted by the majority of oncologists to eradicate the lot.

But here is the problem: chemotherapy medication is only effective for one type and rarely for two or more types of cancer. Furthermore, it is effective only with fifteen to seventeen per cent of the patients.

Also, chemo drugs have toxic side effects that kill more healthy cells than cancer cells and give rise to intolerable suffering on the part of the patient. In the end, surgery, chemo- and radiotherapy, if at all "effective", will prolong the life of the patient only by a few years at best in a tiny number of cases.

Dr. Nicholas Gonzalez, MD, [23] states, "The word 'effective' does not mean cure. [...] To put it in perspective, over 580,000 'effectively treated' cancer patients die[d] in the U.S. [in 2012]. The sobering truth is the cancer industry has only improved the overall cancer death rate by 5% in the last 60+ years. 'Ineffectively treated' is a more accurate and appropriate way to describe the current state of affairs."

Neither should you be fooled by the pictures of smiling adults who suffered "incurable" cancer and were healed against all odds. They are the exception to the rule.

Congratulations to them and hopefully they will lead a very happy and healthy life for many years to come.

Yet, there is no medical professional, oncologist or otherwise, who can say with absolute certainty that it was cut, burn and poison that saved the life of these lucky few patients or the immune system that for unknown reasons kicked in and did the job it is supposed to do.

It has been stated by honest cancer specialists that the conventional treatment palliates, i.e. is at best life extending for a few weeks up to a few years without really improving the cancer patients' quality of life.

Moreover, it is a very expensive procedure and the costs of this treatment have to be borne by health care systems and

---

[23] Dr. Nicholas Gonzalez, MD, 28th Dec. 1947 – 21st July 2015

patient. For this reason alone but also because conventional treatments fail to deliver the desired results, it is understandable that those specialists involved in the research of new, innovative cancer immunotherapy are stating that the conventional cancer treatment is "not working all that well"[24] or "antiquated" [25] and that "the slash, burn and poison approach to cancer has failed"[26].

Even the National Cancer Institute, Baltimore, states on its various very informative pages about cancer treatment that it is not known whether chemotherapy and radiation after surgery helps to keep cancer from recurring. [27] This uncertainty expressed by the world's leading cancer research centre, an authority whose statements can be trusted, is ignored in the tabulation of cancer survival statistics.

Contrary to the opinions expressed by the avant-garde of cancer research, the statistics of agencies around the world claim a significant rise in the number of cancer survivors due to the vast improvements of diagnosis and conventional treatment. One has to read the reports carefully to detect that by "survival" they mean a progression free survival rate of up to five years. They even claim that the number of cancer diagnoses has dropped. But these statistics are based on a standardised mortality rate (SMR) per 100,000. It is a per capita calculation in relation to a nations' total population that contradicts the actual figures of diagnoses and deaths.

A blatant example is the U.S. Centre for Disease Control (CDC) statistic.[28] It claims a decrease in the USA from 171

---

[24] Arthur N. Brodsky, Ph.D. - Cancer Research Institute, New York, NY

[25] Dr. Michael Jensen, founding director of the Ben Towne Center for Childhood Cancer Research, Seattle, WA

[26] Dr. Azra Raza, Professor of Medicine and Director of the MDS Center at Columbia University in New York, NY.

[27] Cancer Treatment, NCI
 (https://www.cancer.gov/about-cancer/treatment)

[28] Expected New Cancer Cases and Deaths in 2020
 (https://www.cdc.gov/cancer/dcpc/research/articles/cancer_2020.htm)

cancer deaths per 100,000 of the population in 2010 to 151 cancer deaths per 100,000 of the population in 2019. Yet, the actual figures in the USA show a rise from 575,000 cancer deaths in 2010 to 630,000 in 2019.

That doesn't look like a decrease, does it now?

A spokeswoman for the Canadian Cancer Society said they're seeing the same trend in Canada. She claims that cancer deaths rates peaked in 1988 and had been decreasing ever since, according to the SMR. "This decrease is largely driven by the progress we've made with lung cancer and prostate cancer in males, breast cancer in females and colorectal cancer in males and females," she said.

An estimated 206,200 new cancer diagnoses and 80,800 cancer deaths occurred in Canada in 2017, according to the society's latest report.[29] Yet, the 2018[30] cancer statistics in Canada showed a rise to 249,077 diagnoses and the number of deaths to 81,378 cases.

The forecast for 2020[31] shows a slight decrease in the number of diagnosed cases of cancer with 225,800 but a significant increase to 83,300 estimated cancer deaths. It is also advisable to take these 2020 figures with a large pinch of salt - they are estimates and will in all likelihood show up dramatically different once the actual figures are tallied.

The evident contradiction in the claims of cancer societies or other official bodies and the actual figures is hidden in the SMR per 100,000 expressed as a ratio that quantifies the death of cancer patients with respect to the general population of a country. The SMR is a formula of the total number of the population divided by 100,000 and using the result as the divisor for the number of cancer deaths. Expressed in actual

---

[29] (https://www.cbc.ca/news/health/cancer-death-rates-canada-us-1.4975106)
[30] WHO Globocan 2018
[31] (https://www.cbc.ca/news/canada/british-columbia/more-cancer-cases-in-canada-2020-1.5482276)

numbers: a population of 37 million divided by 100,000 results in the divisor of 370 for a total number of 85,000 cancer deaths that provides an SMR of 230. To prove that this is just a sick statistician's numbers game let's say the population increased by 2 million immigrants, refugees, and asylum seekers as was recently the case in a few countries and the SMR is suddenly down to 228 showing a 'significant' drop of 1%.

Did the oncologists suddenly become wonder-healers? No, it is just a numbers game that is supposed to make the population believe that conventional cancer treatments are improving, that cancer is under control. Together with the message "Let them smoke pot for recreation" it is reminiscent of Aldous Huxley's dystopian novel "*Brave New World*" where drugs that produce euphoria and hallucination are distributed by the state in order to promote content and social harmony.

The SMR is sophistry at its best - clever but false arguments with the intention of deceiving. It does not show a decrease of cancer diagnoses and deaths but a country's faster rate of population growth than the increase of cases of cancer. The WHO's Global Cancer Observatory predicts an annual increase of cancer diagnoses of up to 4.5 percent from 18.1 million cases in 2018 to between 29 and 37 million over the next twenty years.[32]

What statistics can one believe? As Winston Churchill is supposed to have said, "There are little white lies, big ugly lies, and then there are statistics." How true! Whatever the statistics are trying to make us believe, it is a fact that the global cancer survival rate is not much to trumpet about according to the following sample of global figures.[33]

---

[32] WHO prognosis: Cancer diagnoses will double
RND, 5th March 2020
[33] Globocan 2018 Summary Statistics *(https://gco.iarc.fr/today/ data/factsheets/populations/900-world-fact-sheets.pdf)*

Type of cancer	Diagnosed in 2018	Deaths of patients diagnosed in 2018	% Survivors
Lung	2,093,876	1,761,007	15.9
Breast	2,088,849	626,679	70.0
Colorectal	1,849,518	880,792	52.4
Prostate	1,276,106	358,959	71.9
Stomach	1,033,701	782,685	24.3
Liver	841,080	781,631	7.1
Oesophagus	572,034	508,585	11.1
Pancreas	458,918	432,242	5.8
Others	7,864,875	3,422,447	56.5
Total	18,078,957	9,555,027	47.2

These figures take on a downright sinister appearance when the percentage of deaths of various types of cancer is the guiding factor for each type.

It makes the highly touted much improved treatment of breast and prostate cancer look almost insignificant also in light of over 600,000 women still dying of breast cancer.

Type of cancer	Diagnosed in 2018	Deaths of patients diagnosed in 2018	% Deaths
Pancreas	458,918	432,242	94.2
Liver	841,080	781,631	92.9
Oesophagus	572,034	508,585	88.9
Lung	2,093,876	1,761,007	84.1
Stomach	1,033,701	782,685	75.7
Colorectal	1,849,513	880,792	47.6
Others	7,864,875	3,422,447	43.5
Breast	2,088,849	626,679	30.0
Prostate	1,276,106	358,959	28.1
Total	18,078,957	9,555,027	52.8

The 9,555,027 cancer deaths globally in the year 2018 show that 26,178 people died from cancer every day or 1 person every 3.3 seconds.

Far be it from comparing these figures to the victims of other diseases or afflictions but it must be permitted to raise the question why the media appears to simply accept the vast number of cancer deaths annually as run-of-the-mill while a massive hue and cry is raised over the significantly lower numbers of death due to sudden viral infections or overdosing on drugs.

During the recent corona virus pandemic two positive developments were observed:

- the international collaboration and exchange of virus vaccine research results, and
- the companies Pfizer, GlaxoSmithKline, AstraZeneca, Johnson & Johnson, Merck & Co., Moderna, Novavax, and Sanofi signing the joint statement of a "historic pledge... to uphold the integrity of the scientific process as they work towards potential global regulatory filings and approvals of the first COVID-19 vaccines."[34]

The "historic pledge" reads:

- Always make the safety and well-being of vaccinated individuals our top priority.
- Continue to adhere to high scientific and ethical standards regarding the conduct of clinical trials and the rigor of manufacturing processes.
- Only submit for approval or emergency use authorization after demonstrating safety and efficacy through a Phase 3 clinical study that is designed and conducted to meet requirements of expert regulatory authorities such as FDA.

---

[34] Coronavirus Vaccine Pledge
Chris Smith, 8th Sep. 2020
(https://bgr.com/2020/09/08/coronavirus-vaccine-pledge-phase-3-trials-approval-safety/)

- Work to ensure a sufficient supply and range of vaccine options, including those suitable for global access.
- We believe this pledge will help ensure public confidence in the rigorous scientific and regulatory process by which COVID-19 vaccines are evaluated and may ultimately be approved.

It would not only be most welcome but is urgently needed to see something similar of that scale for the research of cancer immunotherapies. All that is required to issue such a pledge applicable to cancer would be "cancer patients" in place of "vaccinated individuals" and "cancer medications" replacing any reference to "vaccine". Yet, it appears inconceivable that Big Pharma would sign up to "adhere to high scientific and ethical standards regarding the conduct of clinical trials" and "only submit for approval ... after demonstrating safety and efficacy through a Phase 3 clinical study" as regards its cancer medications.

You may well ask why Big Pharma would be unwilling to sign such a pledge. It is due to the inherent difference between a contagious viral pandemic that is of recent origin, and cancer, which is not contagious and has been plaguing humanity forever.

When the viral outbreak became apparent, the fear of becoming infected and dying a horrible death set in among the general public. Consequently, the governments of many countries took rigorous action to contain the virus and invested heavily into R&D of vaccines, which was linked to the demand for a reasonable price per innoculation so it could be covered by the public purse for the entire population.

In step with the government actions was a public outcry against Big Pharma's barely camouflaged efforts to use the pandemic as another form of bilking the public for billions of dollars as was already witnessed with the pricing of allegedly curative "off label" medications. That put practically all pharmaceutical companies involved in the R&D of a corona virus vaccine under enormous public pressure to put public health ahead of its profit maximisation schemes.

All of that - a widespread fear of suffering the disease, governments' rigorous action to help contain the disease, the public purse's massive financial support of R&D, the unequivocal demand for reasonable pricing of medication, and the public outcry against Big Pharma bilking the public and health insurance - it has been missing to the largest extent in regard to finding a cure for cancer.

It would require more than the relatives and caregivers of the over nine million people who die from cancer year after year demonstrating and demanding the governments of their respective countries to support the exploration of every avenue to a cure for cancer, as well as demanding to finally stand up to Big Pharma and take away its pricing policy privilege for the situation to change.

Even such minimal public demand and corresponding government actions are unlikely to happen. Therefore, it is also inconceivable that any pharmaceutical company would feel compelled to sign a similar pledge for cancer medication and the support of R&D of cancer immunotherapy similar to the one signed for virus vaccine.

The Need for a New Approach

A completely new approach, an entirely new way of thinking about cancer treatment and how to eliminate cancer is urgently required. The present division between 'militarist' and 'pacifist' thinking in the field of oncology has to be overcome.

The 'militarists' are those researchers and doctors who insist on the conventional treatment of cut, burn, and poison as the only way to tackle cancer. They want to attack cancer head-on and kill those nasty tumours they can actually see with the 'silver bullet' of costly surgery, chemo- and radiotherapy and declare 'mission accomplished' thus ignoring the billions of cancer cells they can't see that are ready to grow into full-blown cancer tumours.

The 'pacifists' on the other hand want to get to know the "enemy" intimately. They are concerned about these tiny and still invisible cancer cells and try to figure out a way of strengthening the patients' own immune system without over-activating it to avoid a deadly autoimmune response. They research methods of eliminating cancer at its earliest stage without harming healthy tissue and cells.

The 'militarists' are going to be the losers in this battle because their methods have not achieved the desired results in over one hundred years of their conventional cancer treatment. They increased suffering and misery like all militarists do by driving many families of cancer patients into abject poverty with expensive treatments that palliate at best and the prescription of overpriced and generally useless medications.

The 'pacifists' on the other hand have achieved some small yet significant steps towards figuring out how the immune system can do the job it is supposed to do. They have a lot of work ahead of them but will be the winners in the long run.

A Big Hurdle Looms

Many researchers of immunotherapy are investigating the exact nature of what causes every specific type of cancer cell to grow incessantly. Once they have conclusive evidence to that effect, they may then be able to develop a treatment that stops this growth and eliminates all those cancer cells that will develop into full-blown tumours.

It has been claimed by people around the globe, all of them laymen, that is to say they are not professional medics or pharmacologists to the best of anyone's knowledge, that a comprehensive cure for cancer had been developed a long time ago but is suppressed or withheld by the pharma industry. That claim cannot be supported by any evidence and thus it is without merit and not true. Yet, there are several indicators that let Big Pharma appear to be shady operators whose corporate behaviour promotes such claims.

For a start, once a curative therapy is announced and many clinical trials have provided proof that it is what humanity has been hoping for to ring in the end of this scourge, an even bigger hurdle will have to be taken - Big Pharma's resistance to a cure for cancer.

"No way," says Big Pharma! That's crazy, say those who believe Big Pharma or are its shareholders who benefit from the unrelenting drive for profit maximisation! Aren't all pharma companies involved in the research to find a cure as the popular media is obligingly trying to make us believe?

The simple answer to that question is, "No!" And why don't they want to develop a cure, a procedure or treatment that heals patients and makes them healthy? Greed is the short answer to that question. Just ask yourself what annual cancer medication profits pharma companies could report if anyone had developed a comprehensive cure for cancer that actually heals the patient of the disease and is available at a price equivalent to over-the-counter headache medication? Close to zero, zilch, nada...

Pharma companies are in business to make a profit. The pharma industry's sale, it was announced, had achieved annual gross revenue in excess of US$1.7 trillion in 2019 and profits in the hundreds of billions! Why should they want to look for a cure and kill the goose that lays the golden eggs?

The pharma industry is not interested in the research and development of medications that heal patients of whatever ails them. The pharma industry can't make money, never mind a healthy profit with healthy people. Big profits can only be derived from chronically ill patients who continuously have to buy outrageously priced medicine that actually does not cure them.

Let us have a look at how pharma companies arrive at their outrageous prices for their medications.

If Big Pharma and also a lot of small upstarts are to be believed, it is a detailed calculation of the costs of their highly qualified staff, expensive equipment, and many years of research and trials.

However, the truth is far more pathetic, an utter failure in reasoning. For example, when a pharma company charges a million bucks for a one shot treatment, a charge that of late has become quite common, it is often based on the price of a competing drug that is claimed to treat a similar or identical disease.

In short, they don't calculate the price. They look at a competing drug company's charge in the hope that it is the result of a meticulous calculation and consequently charge 'a bit' like a hundred thousand bucks more.

And the worst aspect of this rip-off is that neither company is obliged to provide proof that their respective medications will heal a patient. It is just sufficient for Big Pharma to announce a minor improvement such as stopping the growth of a tumour temporarily to get the authorisation it seeks and charge for that 'new' medicine any price they see fit. That is just one side of the coin of medication pricing.

A short digression into the medical fields of multiple sclerosis, macular degeneration, and corona virus may help understand the questionable business of the pharmaceutical companies' price calculation and how they overcharge, gouge, or, as some people say, 'swindle' patients and health insurance.

The Swiss pharma giant Roche claims to have developed a new drug for multiple sclerosis. It costs €33,000 (US$35,500). Yet, there is a drug on the market for €3000 (US$3,200) that is practically identical.[35]

Roche praises its new drug as an innovation and states that it contains the active substance "Ocrelizumab" - the effect of which is similar to another active ingredient, the 20-year-old substance "Rituximab" that was also developed and manufactured by Roche and has been administered to patients with MS with great success and no serious side effects. The story sounds almost too absurd to be true. But it highlights how pharmaceutical companies gouge patients and health insurance.

Some years ago, a pharmaceutical company came up with a similar idea for the treatment of macular degeneration. A one-time injection with the identical medication rose from €300 (US$320) to over €3,000 (US$3,200). The difference was that the original medication had not been licensed for macular degeneration and was administered "off-label", while the "new" but identical medication under a different name became licensed for such treatment.

That is the crux of the current case: The old drug "Rituximab" was originally developed and approved for the treatment of cancer. By 2000 it had become clear that "Rituximab" was effective for the treatment of MS. However, Roche never requested a formal approval for this treatment.

---

[35] Fragwürdige Geschäfte pharmazeutischer Firmen
Chris Humbs and Ursel Sieber, RBB, 8th Feb. 2018

And thus "Rituximab" had a decisive disadvantage: the patent expired and with it the price monopoly for the manufacturer.

Consequently, Roche focused its activities on a comparable antibody, obtained a new patent for it, and received approval, authorisation, and licensing from the EMA and FDA. Thus, Roche was able to raise the price to a staggering €33,000 (US$35,500).

Roche explained to the German TV-broadcaster ARD's policy magazine *Kontraste*: "The new drug is proven to be the first drug for both forms of MS." Roche claims to have focused on the development of "Ocrelizumab" because it is more effective and more tolerable for long-term use in MS. Since it is a "humanised antibody" there is potentially a "better tolerance" to the human immune system. Also, there are "fewer infusion reactions".

According to the Munich MS specialist Prof. Bernhard Hemmer that is irrelevant in the treatment of patients. He states categorically, "The effect is very similar. Both drugs cause certain cells in the blood to be switched off and both have lasting effects on the inflammatory activity in the brain. Also, the difference in infusion reactions is likely to be of little clinical importance."

Nevertheless, Doctor Hemmer will have to treat his MS patients with the new, much more expensive MS drug. The reason is a mere formal one: since the manufacturer had never applied for a license for the treatment of MS with the old remedy, doctors had to treat their patients with an "off-label" medication. But this is now finished: Since there is an officially approved MS drug on the market, the health insurance companies may only reimburse the approved drug. That's what the law stipulates: German doctors are no longer allowed to prescribe "Rituximab".

The situation is different in Sweden where over 40% of MS patients still get the old drug. Doctors can treat their patients with the trusted and effective remedy. The state allows them to do that and protects them and their patients - not the interests of the pharmaceutical manufacturer.

An even clearer example of the pharmaceutical industry's price calculation was provided by the company Gilead for its Ebola medication "Remdesivir" that allegedly can save lives as an active ingredient against the deadly Covid-19 disease in the corona virus pandemic of 2020.[36]

Medical experts had asked for the six doses of "Remdesivir" that are administered over five days to be offered for US$12.50 or the equivalent of US$2.08 per dose in consideration of the low production cost of the medication that was developed twenty years ago with at least $70 million in U.S. public funding. Also taken into consideration were the facts that administering this drug reduces the mortality rate only by 41.7% and the recovery time by 26.7%, meaning that 58.3% of patients treated with "Remdesivir" still die and 73.3% of patients do not experience a reduction in the recovery time.

Contrary to the medical experts' opinion, unspecified "others" (shareholders and management of Gilead?) stated that a price of US$12,000 for the five-day treatment was fully justified. They based their argument on the alleged benefits of the drug expressed in the number of hospital days saved in the USA. In other words, their price calculation is not based on the production costs and a reasonable profit but on some nebulous claim of alleged cost savings of third parties. Do they actually give a damn about saving lives?

In answer to that question Gilead-CEO Daniel O'Day stated in an open letter, "We are aware of the responsibility that comes with the Remdesivir price." Subsequently, he offered the medication at a 'rock bottom' price of US$2,340 or US$390 per dose for all economically developed countries and some unspecified discount for emerging and developing

---

[36] Hoffnungsträger Remdesivir: Behandlung soll mehr als € 2000 kosten
Christoph Höland, RND, 29th June 2020

countries. That price still amounts to daylight robbery in light of the actual production costs and the yet unproven efficacy of the medication.

Some politicians such as the Representative Katie Porter (D-California) are waking up to the pharma industry's unscrupulous pricing policy. [37] She verbally "eviscerated" Mark Alles, former CEO of the pharma company Celgene, who oversaw the massive price increase from US$215 (€183) to US$763 (€651) for a single pill of the myeloma (bone marrow cancer) and lymphoma (lymph node cancer) drug Revlimid that is supposed to help the immune system *slow down* the tumour growth.

For the required 21 pills of a 28-day cycle the cost rose from US$4,515 (€3,854) to US$16,023 (€13,677) and for one year of treatment from US$54,180 (€46,248) to US$192,276 (€164,246). The cycle has to be repeated until a disease progression or an unacceptable level of toxicity is detected, meaning that the final cost of treatment is indeterminable. That being said, a cancer cure is not on the cards.

Consequently, Ms. Porter asked Mr. Alles if the pill had become more effective and cancer patients needed fewer pills to justify the price increase. His mealy-mouthed response: "Revlimid proved effective in more patients." To what end the pill proved to be effective, he couldn't or wouldn't say. That's when Porter tore Alles apart stating that the only positive effect of the medication was his skill at price gouging to increase his annual US$13 million (€11.1 million) salary by another US$500,000 (€427,000), while the average senior can't even afford to buy one pill.

The digression tells everything you need to know about Big Pharma's pricing policy and how health laws and health

---

[37] Rep. Katie Porter eviscerates pharma CEO with a brutal math lesson about his $13 million salary *Kathryn Krawczyk, 30th Sep. 2020* (*https://www.yahoo.com/news/rep-katie-porter-eviscerates-pharma-205100420.html*)

insurance, albeit unintentionally, support this swindle. It gives an indication how one of the world's largest pharma companies can boast a $22.9 billion turnover and a profit in excess of $14 billion in 2019 with the sale of its ludicrously overpriced cancer medications that do not heal the patients of their cancer and provide at best a life extension of a few days, weeks or months for that matter. The world's pharma companies are thus creating and promoting the impression that they are not engaged in finding a cure for cancer.

Another aspect is their effort to fight a price reduction of their doubtful medication to affordable levels by any means possible. Armies of their lobbyists 'persuade' governments and the respective ministries of health around the world that their medication pricing is perfectly reasonable, and they are believed to the largest extent. Also, they are preventing a further spread of performance linked pricing that was put into law in Italy in 2019. Performance linked pricing means simply that the pharma companies get paid for their medication only once it has been proven to yield the proclaimed effect for each patient taking it and to the extent it actually showed such a therapeutical impact.

As any honest oncologist or cancer specialist, and there are quite a few of them, will admit, the medications prescribed for most of the more than 200 types of cancer, if they have any effect at all, only palliate in up to 17% of cancer patients by providing a life extension of up to three and a half months on average. Well, cheers to that!

Any other industry that provides totally overpriced products with an 83% failure rate and only a partial function of the remaining 17% of just a few months at best would be sued for massive fraud and have to declare bankruptcy! But in the health industry anything goes when the false hope of survival is brought into the game.

A Conspiracy of Silence

The medications and therapies of conventional treatment do not promote a healing process. Even the reports about the number of patients surviving their cancer for some five years after a treatment with radiation and chemotherapy only show that an extension of the patient's life was achieved.

That is not a cure in the sense of the patient being rid of the cancer and not requiring medication any longer or ever again!

Rarely do we come across positive news of someone having been treated successfully for cancer. When it is reported, one learns hardly anything about the treatment the patient received or the procedure or medication that helped to get rid of the cancer tumours except some vague references to surgery and chemo- and radiotherapy.

And one learns even less, if anything at all, about a new discovery or development that actually aims to *heal* cancer patients. We, that is you and I of the general public, appear to be left in the dark about effective and potentially curative cancer treatment and how and where to obtain it.

People who believe that the lack of transparency about cancer treatments is a conspiracy of silence should know that to the largest extent it is true!

The reason one hears so little about a successful treatment is rooted in the fact that every anticancer medication available in our times proves to be effective only for a very limited number of types of cancer and patients. Often the doctors don't know why it works with one patient, shows no effect with another or even kills a patient, or when it resulted in a positive outcome if it wasn't the patient's immune system that caused the apoptosis of cancer cells.

Now imagine what would happen if a medication that was successful with one patient was loudly touted as "The Cancer Killer That Works". Pandemonium would break out among the millions of people diagnosed with cancer every year. They all hope for a quick and certain cure and would be

105

disappointed to learn that the drug is either not suitable for their type of cancer or is effective only for a small percentage of patients suffering from their particular type of cancer. Consequently, it is better to keep anything that is successfully curative a low-key affair for the benefit of keeping the general public quiet and also to avoid the researchers and developers of such a treatment being lambasted as charlatans and frauds by Big Pharma and its obedient sidekicks, the medical journals.

Killing for Profit?

In the course of the panel of Dr. Aseem Malhotra[38], Sir Richard Thompson[39], Prof. Hanno Pijl[40], and Ms. Sarah Macklin[41], presenting their findings of "Big Food and Big Pharma: Killing for Profit?"[42] to the European Parliament, the following statement by Peter Wilmshurst[43], cardiologist, Centre for Evidence Based Medicine, Oxford, UK, was made public:

- Pharma companies and medical device companies have a fiduciary obligation as businesses to make a profit and declare a shareholder dividend by selling their product[s].

- They are not required to sell to consumers (patients and doctors) the best treatment available, though many of us would like that to be the case.

- Real Scandals:

  1. Regulators fail to prevent misconduct by industry, and

---

[38] Aseem Malhotra, Honorary Consultant Cardiologist at Lister Hospital, Stevenage, UK, and Visiting Professor of Evidence Based Medicine at the Bahiana Scholl of Medicine and Public Health, Brazil.
(https://www.rocprivateclinic.com/about-us-london/dr-aseem-malhotra/)

[39] Sir Richard P. H. Thompson, British physician and past president of the Royal College of Physicians, London, UK.

[40] Prof. Hanno Pijl, internist-endocrinologist at the Leiden University Medical Center (LUMC), Netherlands.
(https://hcfseminars.com/hcf-speaker-series/dr-hanno-pijl/)

[41] Sarah Ann Macklin, Nutritionist, London Metropolitan University.
(https://www.sarahannmacklin.com/meet-sarah)

[42] Are Big Food and Big Pharma really killing people for profit globally? Yes, say some of the biggest names in European medicine.
(http://foodmed.net/2018/04/big-food-big-pharma-killing-profit-yes-european-doctors/)

[43] Dr. Peter Wilmshurst, medical doctor and whistle-blower, subject of multiple libel actions by companies whose products he criticised as ineffective.
(https://en.wikipedia.org/wiki/Peter_Wilmshurst)

2. Doctors, institutions, and journals that have responsibilities to patients and scientific integrity collude with industry for financial gain.

Peter Wilmshurst backed up his claim with an evidence submission to the Science and Technology Committee:

- Academic institutions bear responsibility for the pressure to publish for career advancement that can result in research misconduct.

- A record of prominent publications is likely to attract future funding, which institutions demand, and good publicity, which institutions desire.

- Other pressures for misconduct come from the association of academic institutions with industry, when investigators or their institutions hold patents or shares, or they receive payments from industry, so that there is financial pressure to publish research that are profitable for the company and to suppress 'negative' findings.

- Some publications are simply organised criminal activities, which may be at the behest of sponsors, when prominent academics are paid large sums of money by industry to publish false data, or a sponsor may be one of the victims, when payments for conducting research are made to 'investigators', who simply fabricate data.

- Medical journals have financial pressure to publish positive findings of research on drugs and medical devices, because manufacturers buy reprints of the papers for distribution to doctors and pay for advertisements linked to articles favourable to their product.

- Academic institutions conceal research misconduct, destroy evidence, and silence whistle blowers to protect their reputations.

- Journals are reluctant to admit that they publish flawed research, so they commonly refuse to publish failures to replicate.

108

- Fear of libel action contributes to the failure to expose research misconduct.

- Because lenient sanctions are imposed, institutions believe that the misconduct is not very serious, and potential research fraudsters are not deterred.

- I believe that the best way to address the problems of research misconduct would be by making serious forms of research misconduct criminal offences with meaningful sanctions and to have allegations investigated by a statutory independent body with legal powers (comparable to the Health & Safety Executive).

Peter Wilmshurst does not present his claims and evidence from a narrow nationalistic point of view but addresses the underlying global problem of medical research misconduct that is encouraged by academic institutions, supported and financed by the pharma industry, promoted by medical journals, and serves to deceive the general public as well as many medical practitioners.

When it comes to making profits to satisfy their avarice, any academic so inclined, but especially corporate company owners and shareholders will walk over corpses. Proof of these corporate strategies can be found more readily in food manufacturing than in the pharma industry.

Reports are published in the international news about food scandals ranging from fish farms poisoning natural salmon migration streams in Canada and Norway [44], salmonella infected eggs sold in supermarkets, machine separated meat slime offered as pure beef, ham or chicken by ultra-processed food merchants, and high salt and sugar content as well as toxic preservatives in food and drinks.

In summary the question of "Big Food and Big Pharma: Killing for Profit?" was answered with a resounding "Yes!"

---

[44] An Inside Look Into the Fish Industry Reveals Disturbing Facts That Could Threaten Your Health, *Dr. Mercola, 30th April 2016*

Should you have any doubts about this then read the fine print of the ingredients on packaged snack and convenience food. Could you figure out what any of these chemicals are? Ask yourself if you would eat any of those on the list were they offered to you individually.

It is a similar story albeit more difficult to prove with the pharma industry. Anyone who takes a pill to alleviate a headache knows that essentially the pill is poison.

The warnings on the packages state clearly, if you can read the tiny print, that there is a limit to how many of those pills you can take safely and to consult a physician when the pain persists. So far so good. But then the consumer is dumbfounded when his or her favourite over-the-counter pill or powder is accused of containing a known carcinogen and is quickly withdrawn from the market before anyone has the hot idea of launching a multi-million dollar class action suit by those medication consumers that are stricken with cancer.

It becomes a bit more intricate with medications that are supposed to function as anti-cancer therapies. The cancer patient cannot simply buy it in a pharmacy but has to rely on the knowledge and prescription of an oncologist. And that opens up a completely new chapter because in most cases the good doctor can't be quite sure what works for the patient's particular type of cancer and will go ahead with "Let's give it a try and see if it works".

The doctor has to rely on the claims of the manufacturer and the approval and authorisation of the medication by various agencies such as the Food and Drug Administration in the USA and the European Medicines Agency in Europe.

Doctor and patient trust the vast knowledge and most commendable goals of researchers and scientists employed by those agencies. Surely the manufacturers developed and the agencies authorised a medication that will do everything to keep a patient alive and defeat the disease, didn't they?

110

New Cancer Drugs - Expensive and Mostly Useless

In November 2017 the German TV-broadcaster ARD's programme '*Monitor*' shed light on the dirty business of prescribing and selling useless anti-cancer medication [45], which doesn't affect just one patient at a time but potentially millions of cancer patients around the world.

The programme reported that according to the European Medicines Agency (EMA) most 'new' therapies presented for approval are only slightly modified old medications under a new label and, of course, a much higher price.

In a study, the scientists of the EMA, London, UK, systematically evaluated for the first time all the authorisations granted by the EMA between 2009 and 2013 for cancer treatment. They had approved 48 medications for the treatment of 68 types of cancer[46].

The result was sobering: Only half of the approved therapeutic medications were minimally life prolonging or at least offered the patients a bit of relief.

Conversely, half of the approved medications did not meet the most important criterion: they did not offer patients a longer life span or a better quality of life. None of them offered a cure with the aim of healing the patients.

That means that only about 50% of the total of submitted therapies had a minimally 'positive' effect. Nevertheless, all medications were granted approval by the EMA on account of the manufacturers' claim that their medications at least temporarily stopped the spread or reduced the growth of a tumour under lab conditions.

---

[45] Krebsmedikamente ohne Nutzen: zweifelhafter Profit der Pharmaindustrie, *ARD Monitor, 30th Nov. 2017 (WDR, Köln)*

[46] Availability of evidence of benefits on overall survival and quality of life of cancer drugs approved by European Medicines Agency: retrospective cohort study of drug approvals 2009-13 *(http://www.bmj.com/content/359/bmj.j4530)*

However, a temporary stop of the growth or spread of cancer tumours does not mean that the patients will live longer or that the growth and spread of cancer tumours will not accelerate again.

In summary, all therapies were approved, hit the market at prices of up to €232,000 (US$250,000) for a one-year treatment and were prescribed to anyone willing and capable of paying the price.

For several years now, the EMA has been intensifying its efforts to launch new cancer medication more quickly. Such "accelerated approvals" lower the requirements for drug trials. The reasoning: Cancer patients in particular have to have access to new drugs quickly, because there is still an "unmet medical need" for cancer treatment.

In other words, the EMA believed that new drugs were needed urgently. So, it permitted more 'new' drugs, in many cases slightly modified old medications under a new label, to get onto the market, regardless if they were effective therapies or not[47].

The pharma companies pursue this course of relabelling their old products that is bordering on fraudulent practices to justify their demand for higher prices for their 'new' cancer therapies, which exceed by now €100,000 (US$120,000) per patient per year.

It is interesting to note that the Australian Haematologist & Oncologist Prof. Dr. Glenn Begley[48] confirmed what the EMA proved in Europe from the other side of the pond, i.e. North America: A study conducted in the USA in 2012 established that 47 out of 53 alleged landmark preclinical

---

[47] Neue Krebsmedikamente - Teuer und nutzlos
*Ursel Sieber und Lutz Polanz, ARD, Studio WDR Köln, 30th Nov. 2017
(https://www.tagesschau.de/inland/chemotherapie-monitor-101.html)*

[48] Prof. Dr. Glenn Begley, Haematologist/Oncologist, University of Melbourne, Australia
(The Complex Biology of Cancer (Why haven't we cured it yet?)TEDx)

studies of cancer drugs could not be replicated. That shows close to 89% of cancer drugs considered cutting edge developments did not provide the results touted by their manufacturers and were useless.

Prof. Gershom Zajicek, MD,[49] provided the ultimate reality check of the pharma industry's new medications with his analysis of oncology drugs that do not cure cancer.

He cited a study published on 17th June 2017 in *Science Daily* that exposed major flaws in the fast tracking of some drugs. Stringent clinical evidence of their benefits was not issued and many patients with serious illnesses are being treated with questionable drugs. These drugs were given accelerated approval by the FDA without any strong clinical evaluation.

Zajicek cited data manipulation with surrogate endpoints, the manipulation of clinical trial results, and the FDA's approval of flawed cancer drugs. Most contemporary approvals of new cancer drugs are made on the basis of the surrogate endpoint, i.e. the progression free survival (PFS) from the start of remission to the recurrence of cancer.

The results suggest that the FDA is approving costly, toxic drugs that do not improve the patients' survival. During the study period of 2010 to 2012, 36 of 54 contemporary cancer drug approvals (67%) were made on the basis of the surrogate endpoint. 31 of these approvals had no known effects on the observed survival or failed to show any gains in survival.

He explained what the surrogate fallacy is about: A patient is diagnosed with cancer and, for example, treated with surgery to remove a tumour. The patient feels healthy but the cancer recurs and ultimately the patient dies.

---

[49] Most new Oncology Drugs do not cure Cancer
Gershom Zajicek, M.D., Professor of Experimental Medicine and Cancer Research, Faculty of Medicine, Hebrew University of Jerusalem

Cancer recurrence is the surrogate endpoint and death is the clinical endpoint. The period from the start of remission until the cancer recurs is the progression free survival (PFS) while the period from recurrence until death is the observed survival (OS). He proved with a group of 100 patients that PFS does not predict OS. Yet the FDA claims that the surrogate endpoint, the recurrence of cancer, is used because the clinical endpoint might take a very long time to study and claims that surrogate PFS distribution correlates with and predicts OS distribution. That is a false assumption, a fallacy.

Yet, the FDA insists on surrogate endpoints that have undergone this testing. They are accepted, established, or validated surrogate endpoints, and are accepted by the FDA as proof of benefit. Between 2010 and 2012 the FDA approved 45% of new drugs on the basis of the surrogate endpoint.

The root of this fallacy is that PFS refers to the recurrence of cancer, while OS refers to the death of the patient. The entire procedure starts with the diagnosis, followed by therapy and remission (PFS), then the recurrence and ultimately the diagnosis of death (OS). The remission establishes the PFS but as is often claimed it does not mean the patient is cured.

On the other hand the OS is final since it is the diagnosis of death. Only the OS provides conclusive evidence that a drug prolonged survival and its effectiveness for remission. The PFS does not prove prolonged survival. In short: Symptom elimination does not assure a cure.

Surrogate distribution is unreliable. It doesn't distinguish between drugs that provide a benefit and those that don't. That is the reason why so many drugs appear on the market today that are extremely toxic and do not provide a cure.

Since all Big Pharma companies operate globally, it is likely that the same companies are pushing their useless drugs around the globe based on the FDA's approval.

Making the already gloomy impression of Big Pharma even gloomier is the fact that they spend twice as much on

114

marketing their dubious products than on research and development of truly innovative cancer medications.

Here is a suggestion for Big Pharma to improve its image: Shift just 25% of your marketing budget for dodgy products to the R&D of cancer medications that actually prolong life, improve the patients' quality of life and in the best case provide a cure. Admittedly, you would have a few billion dollars less to spend on gifts and payments to corruptible doctors and institutions but you could actually gain the trust of the public by showing that you are concerned about patient care and you would still make a whopping profit. Should you shift 50% of your marketing budget to research and development, it would make your howling and teeth chattering about the enormous R&D costs of your cancer medications a bit more believable.

But fat chance of that ever coming to pass as long as the pharma companies' owners and shareholders will dictate that the rise in share prices and dividend payments are far more important than developing cancer medications that actually heal patients of their disease.

That was put into perspective with an article of the American Social Security Network[50] that addressed the lack of vaccine development specifically but is valid for R&D of all medications. The report stated what is true for the USA but after a closer look turns out to be just as applicable in most other countries that are home to Big Pharma, namely that the pharma industry actually does very little research.

It states that the riskiest and most crucial research and development of medications is done by universities and thus funded by the taxpayers. In the USA the funding of basic science research is funnelled through the National Institute of Health (NIH) often to the tune of 100% and in Europe the total cost including late stage clinical trials is covered 50% to 75%

---

[50] Alex Lawson, Chairman of the Social Security Network,
People's Action Blog, 25th March 2020

with grants from cancer care organisations that receive their money from governments, i.e. the taxpayers.

Big Pharma acquires the patent monopolies for a nominal fee to produce the drugs and uses this privilege to charge whatever price it sees fit to achieve profit maximisation. Legislation is required to revoke such privilege and allow generic competition to drive down prices when Big Pharma abuses its monopoly with outrageous medication pricing.

Furthermore, the manufacturing of drugs, as has been demanded in several European countries, should be in the public domain with no patent monopolies but immediate generic production of the approved drugs that provided proof of their efficacy in a randomised empirical clinical trial. That would be a step in the right direction because the reduction of the cost of medication would benefit the health insurance systems and hence the general public. Also, it would assure the FDA and EMA of a stop to Big Pharma's fudging of the alleged efficacy of 'new' drugs and the rebranding of old drugs with minimal changes into 'new' drugs.

Any hospital or doctor around the world who wishes to obtain information [51] about the EMA's authorisations and approved medications' level of efficacy or lack of it can do so through the Internet or by direct inquiry.

It is fair to assume that most doctors could find out that the cancer therapies they want to or do prescribe are in the majority useless, do not prolong life and certainly do not eradicate cancer cells, which raises the suspicion of collusion of doctors, pharmacies, and Big Pharma.

Such collusion is under investigation in Europe. It involves kickbacks of the happy threesome of a doctor prescribing a particular pharma company's overpriced medicines that can only be obtained at a specific pharmacy.

---

[51] European Medicines Agency:
"Send a question via our website: www.ema.europa.eu/contact"

The final results of this investigation are not yet in although meetings of the three parties in question were recorded with hidden cameras. It revealed the strenuous efforts to cover up the dirty business with creative bookkeeping and getting banks and insurance companies involved to help cover the tracks.

Not far behind in the 'Department of Dubious Behaviour' are some university hospitals. A blatant example were two researchers from a university hospital in Switzerland who boasted that they 'can' engineer the immune system, 'can' engineer T-cells from scratch that recognise cancer, and 'can' do all sorts of wonderful things with their innovative radio-oncology - but they can't talk about any of it because it is, of course, top secret.

Question is: if they 'can' do all that, why don't they do it and show that they can heal at least a few of the millions of people diagnosed with cancer? What are they waiting for? Does somebody have to drop a couple of billion bucks into their private bank accounts in some tax haven for them to willingly give up their top secret? Or are these researchers only boasting?

One will never find out if they were merely looking for their fifteen minutes of fame.

An Investigation of Corruption and Fraud

Fraudulent activities involving pharma companies, doctors, and institutions are indeed a global menace as it was uncovered by a team of investigative journalist of the very respected and highly reputable newspaper 'Zeit' from Hamburg, Germany[52].

It was reported in the paper and on TV in December 2019, that their research had uncovered a multi-million euro fraud scheme with cancer drug prescriptions by three pharmacists. Their scheme was made possible with the financial support of investors from the UK, Switzerland, the USA, and Canada.

The three pharmacists who are the alleged instigators of the fraudulent scheme had thrown their lot together and founded a company that obtained a licence to manufacture cancer drug infusions.

In order to make their newly founded company commercially successful they purchased doctors' practices at a multiple of the usual market price with the financial assistance of international investors. In turn they employed the doctors of the practices now owned by the company at a minimal salary but huge bonuses for the exclusive prescription of the three pharmacists' cancer drug infusions.

For this scheme to be profitable, the doctors had to prescribe the company's infusions. Consequently, the doctors put profit ahead of patient care to increase their own as well as the company's profits by prescribing vast numbers of excessively expensive infusion therapies that are not medically necessary or beneficial to the patients.

---

[52] Firma soll Millionenbetrug mit Krebsmedikamenten organisiert haben
(https://www.zeit.de/gesellschaft/zeitgeschehen/2019-12/grossrazzia-hamburg-krebsmedikamente-betrug-enthuellung) and
Wie man sich einen Onkologen kauft
(https://www.zeit.de/gesellschaft/zeitgeschehen/2019-12/krebsmedikamente-zytoservice-betrug-onkologen-gesetzesluecke-hamburg)

Such activity contradicts best practice of patient safety and contravenes the respective laws of the European Union.

The three pharmacists founded a nebulous network of companies in Hamburg, Luxemburg, and the Channel Island of Jersey to avoid prosecution or at least make their activities almost untraceable. These companies own each other with an intricate setup of share-holding. In addition, the pharmacists purchased a bankrupt private district clinic in Hamburg.

The clinic, without an oncology department, only fifteen beds, and presumably no patients, enabled them pro forma to establish medical provision centres, which only non-profit organisations and hospitals are permitted to do in Europe.

Thus, they set up an operational trail of the prescriptions being handed by the doctor to a medical provision centre that passed it on to the district clinic that submitted it to the holding company in Hamburg that gave it to the cancer drug infusion laboratory.

Thereby they created a safe distance between the doctors writing prescription and their cancer drug infusion manufacturing facility that would obscure any obvious link between the doctors and the laboratory.

They raked in multi-million-euro profits by charging the prescriptions to health insurance companies. Small wonder that even such otherwise quite honourable institutions like the Alberta Teachers Retirement Fund in Canada had got wind of a quick buck to be made, probably persuaded by its investment advisers that it was okay to invest heavily in a dodgy operation in a foreign country.

Alas all the involved parties had made their calculations without consideration for the small cancer drug infusion manufacturers who before that business was started had supplied the now enslaved doctors with their product and suddenly were given no more orders.

Quite understandably pissed off about being cut out of the lucrative local drug supply market and in some cases having

119

to declare bankruptcy, they started the ball rolling. They informed the team of investigative journalists who needed more than a year of persistent inquiries to unravel the intricate network of alleged fraud, corruption, and contravening against best practice of patient safety. They presented their findings to the state prosecutor of the city-state of Hamburg who launched an investigative process into fraud and to help resolve fundamental health service corruption issues.

Don't you wish there were many more of those gutsy investigative journalists active around the world like this team[53] from Hamburg? It is high time to put an end to massive rip-off schemes with excessively priced anti-cancer medications that mostly don't work, corruption in the medical services sector, and to put fraudulent pharmacists and doctors who put their greed ahead of patient care out of business and behind bars.

---

[53] Robert Bongen, Oliver Hollenstein, Oliver Schröm, and Caroline Walter

Corruption and Fraud is Widespread

In the medical profession, especially in the field of oncology, it should not come as a surprise that corruption and fraud is almost universal.

Big Pharma with its multi-billion-dollar profits can easily afford to keep doctors toeing the line and on their toes. Doctors and institutes rely on the largesse of Big Pharma ladling out billions of dollars for 'research'. As a result, the suspicion of funny business going on raises its ugly head.

A report in the publication "The Truth About Cancer"[54] cites a survey of 11.5 million public records in the U.S. that provides proof of nearly three out of four doctors having direct financial ties to drug companies and medical equipment manufacturers to the tune of US$8.4 billion in gifts and payments over four years.

Quote: "Dr. Aaron S. Kesselheim [55], a professor of medicine at Harvard Medical School and lead author of the survey, says this may be influencing doctors' behavior."

You don't say!

And this reprehensible activity is by no means limited to the USA. It is a problem of a vast number of doctors and institutions being deep in the pockets of Big Pharma in many countries around the world.

This was confirmed by a report on German TV's news broadcast under the headline "When doctors let themselves be seduced"[56]. It showed that in Germany some 18,500 doctors

---

[54] Report: Most Doctors Receive Gifts from Big Pharma
Ty Bollinger, 8th Nov. 2018
(https://thetruthaboutcancer.com/gifts-big-pharma/)
[55] Aaron S. Kesselheim, M.D., J.D., M.P.H., Harvard Medical School
(https://bioethics.hms.harvard.edu/ faculty-staff/aaron-seth-kesselheim)
[56] Wenn sich Ärzte verführen lassen
Christian Baars und Markus Grill, NDR/WDR, 27th June 2020
(https://www.tagesschau.de/investigativ/ndr-wdr/anwendungsbeobachtungen-123.html)

were reported to the German Federal Association of Statutory Health Insurance Physicians. They received so-called "expense allowances" of between €140 (US$157) and €1437 (US$1612) per patient for what is nicely circumscribed as "non-interventional post-marketing studies" (NIPMS). One pharmaceutical company alone distributed around €100 million (US$112.2 million) a year to doctors in Germany for what is supposed to be an application observation of particular drugs. Doctors are paid to allegedly observe and document how well their patients tolerate these drugs. Experts state that these "studies" are scientifically worthless because there is no control group.

The NIPMS have been classified as a form of "legal corruption". The participating doctors prescribe the medications 7 to 8 percent more often than alternative medicine for the same indications. It is influenced by the expense allowances they receive with the aim of marketing the drug. It poses a risk for the patients since side effects are not noted in an observation of tolerance.

The report is largely based on a two-year examination of 7,000 doctors by a group of researchers led by the two physicians Cora Koch of Freiburg University Hospital and Klaus Lieb from Mainz University Hospital that was published in the renowned US journal "PLOS Medicine"[57].

For the purpose of the examination they investigated two groups: one of doctors participating in the application observation of particular drugs and a control group of doctors who did not participate. Thus, they provided proof that the

---

[57] Impact of physicians' participation in non-interventional post-marketing studies on their prescription habits: A retrospective 2-armed cohort study in Germany
Cora Koch, Jörn Schleeff, Franka Techen, Daniel Wollschläger, Gisela Schott, Ralf Kölbel, Klaus Lieb, 26th June 2020,
https://doi.org/10.1371/journal.pmed.1003151
(https://journals.plos.org/plosmedicine/article?id=10.1371/journal.pmed.1003 151)

participating doctors prescribed the medications in question seven to eight percent more often than the other doctors during the NIPMS and the year thereafter and established the influence of marketing the drug, which adds to the large body of evidence indicating that lucrative interaction between physicians and the pharmaceutical industry influence physician behaviour.

The German research group came to the same conclusion as Dr. Kesselheim in the USA despite their different methodology in the approach to the investigation. In view of the disparate health care systems of the two countries, it is safe to surmise that the problem of doctors and institutions deep in the pockets of the pharmaceutical industry is global and would be uncovered in other countries if investigated.

Further proof[58] of this nefarious activity was provided by the U.S. Justice Department's $678 million settlement with the pharma giant Novartis in July 2020 over improper inducements it made to doctors to prescribe the company's drugs. Novartis increased annual profits by at least $40 million as a result of the conduct, money that was paid by federal health care programs, the government said.

"For a decade, Novartis spent hundreds of millions of dollars on so-called speaker programs, including speaking fees, under the guise of providing educational content, when in fact the events served as nothing more than a means to provide bribes to get doctors to prescribe Novartis's drugs," said Audrey Strauss, the acting U.S. attorney for southern New York (SDNY), whose office prosecuted the case.

The case came to light when Oswald Bilotta, a Novartis sales representative for the eastern end of Long Island, New York, filed a suit in January 2011 under the False Claims Act, detailing remuneration to physicians, such as lavish dinners at

---

[58] It was his dream job. He never thought he'd be bribing doctors and wearing a wire for the feds.

NBC News, Gretchen Morgenson and Kit Ramgopal, 7th July 2020

restaurants, costly tickets to sporting events and entertainment, including a trip to a Manhattan strip club, gift cards, and catering for events of doctors' children, such as graduations or bar mitzvahs. The U.S. government and New York state took up his case in 2013. It covers activities of Novartis from January 2002 until November 2011 and involved kickbacks resulting in higher health care costs, overuse of drugs or services, and improper patient steering. Over the period, one doctor received over $320,000 in honoraria and wrote more than 8,000 prescriptions for the company's drugs, the government said.

It must be absolutely infuriating for the doctors and institutions who do not accept bribes in the form of 'gifts' or 'kickbacks' to have their reputation dragged through the mud by their utterly corruptible peers who in all likelihood do not consider patient care their top priority.

Underscoring the point of medical professionals making loads of money by being corruptible is the story of a teacher asking his tenth grade pupils if they had given any thought to the profession they wanted to pursue as adults. One of the boys jumped up and sounded off that he wanted to be a doctor. The teacher praised the boy for his evidently humanistic goal of wanting to heal the sick to which the boy replied, "Whatever gives you that idea? No way! I want to become a doctor to rake in oodles of money, become filthy rich, and retire before I'm forty." Point taken...

So, don't be surprised, wherever you may reside on our blue planet, when an oncologist eagerly recommends or even prescribes a medication that costs over a hundred thousand dollars for a year's treatment and will at best extend the patient's life only by a few weeks or months.

That begs the question how a doctor, cancer specialist or not, can in all conscience prescribe a medication that doesn't have any life-prolonging or curative effect but lets the patient and his family potentially descend into abject poverty?

Also, don't be flabbergasted when the oncologist scoffs at the proven and many times replicated efficacy of a generic adjunct medication after a cursory glance at the papers of a scientific report and deposits it in the nearest waste bin.

The documents and scientific reports of *in vitro* and *in vivo* trials of adjunct as well as adjuvant medication and its application that provide proof of its effectiveness are audaciously ignored or even ridiculed, especially when they are affordable.

Many other reports of successful treatments with medication from foreign countries[59] suffer the same fate. This attitude varies by degree from country to country but is encountered globally.

---

[59] Made in Cuba: A cancer treatment with less toxic side effects
*Tan Shiow Chin, The Star (Malaysia), 18th Oct. 2017
(https://www.star2.com/health/wellness/2017/10/18/cuban-cancer-treatment-success-story/)*

The Media Needs to Differentiate

Anything ingested or inhaled in excess is deadly. That is a self-evident truth and applies equally to vital, innocuous substances such as water and air as well as medications and known toxins.

However, a vast number of toxins administered in miniscule amounts can have a therapeutic effect and save lives. Therefore, one should differentiate between a quantity that kills and one that can save a life.

Yet, when it comes to reports and documentaries about opioids such differentiation appears to be overlooked. At least one will be very hard pressed to find any references to the actual quantity of an opioid that kills or, for that matter, the quantity in milligrammes of a specific opioid with the potential or proven therapeutic effect that saves a life.

The opioid crisis has received a lot of publicity over the past few years due to the large increase in the number of people dying from an overdose of heroin or fentanyl. That is indeed a very tragic development.

Pharma companies were identified as the culprits for having caused the outbreak of the crisis. One company, Purdue Pharma claimed that their semi-synthetic opioid OxyContin was the most effective pain management medication and not addictive. Hence, it became a commonly prescribed medication in the USA with more than 1.5 million prescriptions a year. Purdue had to declare bankruptcy when it became embroiled in multibillion-dollar settlement negotiations over its alleged culpability in the opioid crisis and the U.S. Justice Department was seeking $18.1 billion in criminal and civil penalties.[60]

---

[60] Justice Department Seeks Billions In Penalties From OxyContin Maker Purdue Pharma, *Palash Ghosh, 8th May 2020*
(*https://www.ibtimes.com/justice-department-seeks-billions-penalties-oxycontin-maker-purdue-pharma-3023091*)

Many doctors still prescribe this generic painkiller even for ailments that could be treated more effectively with acupuncture or physiotherapy. But it is so much easier and quicker for a doctor to prescribe a pill than to determine which alternative treatment would be better, find an acupuncturist or a physiotherapist, and write a referral.

Once the patients can't afford the expensive prescription medication any longer, the alternative is the street dealer offering heroin and fentanyl at much lower prices. Only very few addicts manage to get off this slippery slope with the help of families, friends, or in rehabilitation centres.

In regard to cancer it would be very helpful for patients as well as the medical practitioners treating them if producers of documentaries and reporters of news on the Internet, TV, the radio and printed media would finally become aware of and begin to differentiate between the quantity of opioids that kills and the quantity that has been proven to provide a cure in the best case or help as an adjunct or adjuvant in the apoptosis of cancer tumours and many other medical problems and illnesses especially mental disorders.

Less than four years before the time of this writing, I still had absolute faith in the medical profession and the pharmaceutical industry based on what I had read, heard and seen in the media. What else was I supposed to believe? I'm not a medical practitioner. Little did I know then that most of what one gleans from the media about the fantastic efficacy of the latest and totally new cancer medication and treatment is unadulterated bullshit! Mostly it amounts to the uncritical regurgitation of the pharma companies' or researchers' press releases by unqualified hacks as well as the jingoistic hyperbole of nationalistic yahoos who wish to convince their compatriots and the world that their country is at the cutting edge of cancer research.

It could be said that one shouldn't believe everything that is reported and not be so damn gullible. That may be true, but then, what should one believe? Isn't journalism in all its forms supposed to be based on thorough investigation and critical assessment of the facts? Alas, that may have been the case in the past but it doesn't apply any longer especially when it comes to reporting pharmaceutical discoveries that are proclaimed to be of promise in treating cancer.

It takes time and comparative and critical reading, watching, and listening to separate the wheat from the chaff of health reports. What hits one first is the extensive use of the conditional such as should, could, would, might, etc. in regard to the anticipated efficacy of a substance still under investigation. When the conditional is not used, it is usually in conjunction with the verb 'promising' as regard medical discoveries and research.

What does that actually mean that a discovery is 'promising'? Generally, it means absolutely nothing. In fact, often it refers to the theory of some researcher who insists that because his or her research has shown some result in lab tests involving petri dishes and perhaps mice that the same results can be achieved in the treatment of humans.

What one does not read or hear is the phrase 'it is curative' or that it heals cancer patients.

It would be interesting to see some reliable data of how many of those 'promising' discoveries and developments over the past forty or fifty years have never been heard of again or were condemned outright to be detrimental to the patients who took it in good faith, resulted in their palliative and hospice care, and early death.

Palliative & Hospice Care

Once a person is diagnosed with cancer, doctors will fall back on wanting to prescribe some expensive therapy as a first course of action. Often they do that against better knowledge of the therapies' lack of efficacy. Thus, they create the impression of being indentured to their feudal master - Big Pharma.

When the therapy fails to show positive results and conventional measures such as surgery, chemo- and radiotherapy have been tried and failed or were ruled out, the terms palliative and hospice care are bandied about without any specific clarification of what that implies.

The dictionary definition of 'palliative' is a "treatment or medicine relieving pain or alleviating a problem without dealing with the underlying cause". It is derived from the Latin verb *palliare*, which means "to cloak", "to cover up".

It raises the question, what is meant to be cloaked or covered up - the patient's suffering, the medics' inability or unwillingness to deal with the underlying cause of the patient's illness, their lack of knowledge, or their bias? Or is it a case of the principal aphorism of modern medicine, "*primum non nocere*" (Latin for "first, do no harm")? It implies that it is better not to do anything that might risk doing more harm than good, which is ludicrous when a patient is given only a few days, weeks, or months to live.

That, of course, lends itself marvellously as a cover for a medic who either lacks knowledge of or is biased against the successful treatment of cancer that was achieved in foreign countries, especially when such treatment has not been approved on his home turf.

It will leave a whole slew of avenues of cancer treatment unexplored with the excuse that such nationally unapproved treatment could cause more harm than good and leaves those doctors who would be willing to explore "unapproved treatments" at the mercy of a bunch of bureaucrats in their respective health services who most likely don't know anything or care very little about individual patients and opens the path to palliative care as the only alternative.

Palliative care starts in an outpatient setting usually followed by the inpatient continuation of hospice care.

A hospice (from Latin *hospitium*, meaning "hospitality" or "hostel") is a facility of terminal care. It is mostly in a residential setting with only a few beds at its disposal.

In some countries a team of specialists works together with the primary caregiver and family doctor to give support, while in many other countries a palliative care specialist may rely on the assistance of a nurse but forbids any interference from family doctor or caregiver, e.g. in Canada according to my experience.

Palliative care has no curative intent in most of the world. Yet, in several European countries and the USA it is often dispensed along with curative therapies and medications. Thus, the general term 'Palliative Care' by itself is misleading. It should be replaced by the more specific terms 'Palliative Curative Therapy' and 'Palliative Non-curative Therapy', respectively, when the treatment is meant to have a curative intent or not.

The Word Heath Organisation (WHO) should be at the forefront of this change in terminology because it is the organisation with global outreach and mostly referred to for clarification of terms. It states in its "Definition of Palliative Care" that it is "an approach that improves the quality of life of patients and their families facing the problems associated with life-threatening illness, through the prevention and relief of suffering by means of early identification and impeccable assessment and treatment of pain and other problems, physical, psychosocial and spiritual".[61]

---

[61] Palliative Care - Key facts
   (https://www.who.int/news-room/fact-sheets/detail/palliative-care)

That WHO definition of palliative care lends itself for a good belly laugh. While early identification and impeccable assessment of illness is certainly not part of palliative care, the rest of the statement only applies in a perfect world.

In reality it should differentiate between curative and non-curative palliative therapies that have disparate outcomes due to their aims. While the curative therapy intends to achieve healing and survival by all medical means possible, the non-curative therapy gives up on healing and puts the patient in a drug-induced and hopefully pain-free end of life. Thus, the non-curative therapy does not improve the quality of life within the confines of the hospice and is not based on impeccable assessment of pain and problems.

The term 'palliative care' was coined by Dr. Balfour Mount[62]. He didn't think the term 'hospice' was appropriate because in French it has the connotation of poorhouse. He began to provide a service for terminally ill patients in the francophone province of Québec, Canada, after he had observed hospice services in Britain.

Dr. Mount intended to achieve with his introduction of palliative care in Canada a facility to take care of the terminally ill who have no caregiver or family able to support them and are indeed at the end of their life.

What it has become in the form of the modern-day hospice in Canada is a facility that provides only palliative non-curative therapy, a catchall for many patients who should be admitted to an acute care ward of a hospital where every effort should be made to save their life.

Instead, doctors who have given up on those patients, don't want to treat them any longer or are hindered by bureaucracy to administer life-saving medication, shuffle them off to a

---

[62] The father of palliative care in Canada, physician Balfour Mount on the legacy of Cicely Saunders, the start of palliative care, and the true meaning of medical aid in dying
(https://www.mcgill.ca/palliativecare/portraits-0/balfour-mount)

hospice to be given end-of-life treatment with useless analgesics like fentanyl that literally assure a quick death.

And the worst aspect of this patient treatment is the fact that families and caregivers are not properly informed of a hospice providing palliative non-curative therapy that won't allow any interference of family and caregiver or palliative curative therapy that gives the patient as well as family and caregiver a say in what medication should be administered and a chance for survival.

Would patient, family, or caregiver agree to a palliative non-curative therapy, if it were stated clearly by the doctor? Depending on the age and the physical condition of the patient, the family might agree to assure a painless end of life. But in the case of a patient in otherwise fair physical condition besides the actual illness and when available treatments have not been considered or administered for whatever reason, the family or caregiver would not agree to have the patient subjected to a non-curative therapy until every avenue of a cure has been exhausted.

In some countries, the USA for example, hospice care includes palliative curative therapy by administering a range of life extending and even curative medications, monitoring equipment, and around-the-clock access to care where in all nursing and medical acts the patient's will comes first.

That means the medical staff has to abide by the patient's will and cannot follow the aphorism of "*primum non nocere*" due to a lack of medical knowledge or unfounded fears of addiction when a patient requests to be treated with a specific medication that fits into the overall curative therapy or does not want to have a specific medicine administered. And that makes sense in palliative care.

The prerequisite for admission to an inpatient hospice in most countries is that the patient suffers from an incurable disease that generally excludes a cure and will lead to death in the foreseeable future.

That is a loaded precondition. It raises the question of who decides that a disease excludes a cure? What is meant by death in the foreseeable future?

It is foreseeable after all that every human being, every living organism will die eventually. So, who decides that someone should be admitted to a hospice? Well, for example in Canada that decision is based merely on the verbal opinion of a general practitioner or specialist - at least in my experience.

Compare that to the requirements in France, Germany, and several other European countries where the admission to inpatient hospice care has to be *prescribed* by a doctor.

The prescription must be backed up by the documented diagnosis, a succinct prognosis, and further details such as distressing symptoms that require special care and attention.

According to law the doctor has to issue a complete medical certificate that clearly establishes and documents the need for full-time inpatient hospice care.

Isn't that how it should be in the case of life and death?

One Crisis Noted - Another Practically Ignored

The media made the world aware of the 'Opioid Crisis' when it was thought that it was dealing with a single enemy, namely the clear and present danger of opioids.

Yet, first line drug combatants such as drug agencies, police chiefs, and the mayors of several metropolitan cities were ignored. They had expressed the opinion since the 1970s that it is ludicrous to declare a drug an enemy and a war on drugs as long as there is something fundamentally wrong with those societies most severely affected by a crisis of people dying from an opioid overdose.

The media also paid little attention to a very important factoid: addicts take 600mg of opioids or more a day to satisfy their cravings. Any doctor worth his or her salt knows that the level of life-threatening opioid toxicity begins at 50mg. No wonder so many addicts die from an overdose.

The fact that thousands of people addicted to drugs die every year from an opioid overdose is indeed lamentable and atrocious. It is also preventable. But our societies do not provide the perspective and help needed by millions of people, especially young people, to prevent them from going down the slippery slope of drug consumption.

In other words, the enemy is not the opioid - it is us!

But our societies are so focused on the accumulation of money and the acquisition of material things that scant attention is paid to social problems.

That is probably the reason why nobody dares to address a 'Cancer Crisis'. Cancer isn't a single, clearly identifiable 'enemy'. It is a very complex disease and encountered in a vast range of afflictions.

Not thousands, but millions of people are diagnosed with cancer every year and die from it, which appears to be taken as par for the course. At least one doesn't hear or read anything about a 'Cancer Crisis' or 'Cancer Emergency'. Yet with 9 million people dying from cancer a year at present and much more to come, wouldn't it be justified to address it as such?

The World Health Organisation (WHO) forecast in 2010 that globally some 15 million new cases of cancer would be diagnosed in the year 2020. Well, the WHO low-balled their estimates quite evidently because already in 2019 more than 18.5 million people were diagnosed with cancer.

Accordingly, the WHO has updated its forecast and predicts that between 29 and 37 million people will be diagnosed with cancer globally by the year 2040. That is some twenty years to go and appears to be low-balled again in view of the annual increases over the past twenty years.

This increase points to something seriously wrong with the societies, particularly those of countries considered to be economic 'powerhouses' and several so-called emerging nations that are home to the mega-corporations hailed for their prowess and economic success but rarely held accountable in all seriousness for the damage they do to the environment and public health.

Cancer societies around the world publish annual reports about cancer and the over 200 identified types of the disease, as well as the increase of people diagnosed with cancer, and, naturally, how to prevent getting full-blown cancer.

The major topic dealing with cancer prevention is the assessment of lifestyles, which essentially results in blaming the persons diagnosed with cancer for getting the disease.

As an aside: blaming the cancer victims for getting the disease was the favourite accusation of the Nazis [63] in Germany. Not much has changed since the 1930s in this regard, has it?

The often quite simplistic warnings are summarised in alcohol and tobacco consumption, obesity, a lack of physical

---

[63] So hat sich der Umgang mit der Krankheit gewandelt
RND, Kristian Teetz, 12th March 2020

exercise, taking excessive amounts of prescription or over-the-counter drugs, and eating unhealthy food.

In short, the cancer victims are blamed for getting cancer that could be prevented with a healthy lifestyle.

What has never been investigated to the best of anyone's knowledge are people who consume alcohol and smoke tobacco products, are overweight and sit quietly in a corner until the urge to exercise subsides, eat only junk food, pop headache pills by the handful to treat their hangovers, and never get cancer.

A prime candidate would have been the writer Kurt Vonnegut[64] who said that he would sue the makers of his favourite brand of cigarettes he had been smoking since he was twelve or fourteen years old for false advertising. "And do you know why?" he said. "Because I'm 83 years old. The lying bastards! On the package [they] promised to kill me."

Another candidate for such research would have been the former German chancellor Helmut Schmidt.[65] He enjoyed beer or wine with every meal (except breakfast) and chain-smoked until the day he died of natural causes at the ripe old age of 96. Stuff that in your pipe and smoke it!

These examples of heavy smokers into old age should not be understood as a defence of smoking. The consumption of tobacco in any form is unhealthy. Full stop. Yet, it should be noted that it is not just the tobacco leaf that is the culprit of causing diseases but the chemicals that are added by the manufacturers of tobacco products to make them more addictive. And that sheds once more a dubious light on governments that rake in billions of tobacco tax dollars and

---

[64] Interview Rolling Stone Magazine 2006, Kurt Vonnegut, Writer of 14 novels, short-story collections, plays, and works of non-fiction   11th Nov. 1922 - 04th Nov. 2007

[65] Helmut Schmidt, Chancellor of the Federal Republic of Germany from 1974 to 1982, 23rd Dec. 1918 – 10th Nov. 2015

refuse to pass any legislation to ban and heavily penalise the drenching of tobacco with addictive substances. Without being facetious it can be presumed that the governments also refuse to do so because smokers generally die earlier than non-smokers and thus save the governments billions of dollars in old age pension and health care payments.

So, why are there no investigations of people with outrageously unhealthy lifestyles that never get cancer? Are the doctors and health care advocates afraid of finding something that will toss all their assumptions about a healthy lifestyle preventing cancer into a cocked hat?

Also, what is given scant attention and rarely investigated is the exposure to pathogens such as bacteria, viruses, and microorganisms, carcinogenic chemicals such as fertilisers, herbicides and insecticides, ultraviolet light and ionising radiation, and environmental pollutants such as dioxides and the radioactive gas radon. Even the healthiest of lifestyles cannot prevent the exposure to any of these cancer-causing substances that are normally suffered at the place of work, the outdoors, or in the home environment.

Furthermore, no explanation is given, not a word is lost on people with a healthy lifestyle who have no genetic disposition or family history of cancer, still get the disease, and die from it. That might be only a very small percentage of the millions of people diagnosed with cancer every year. Still, every year thousands of children of families who care for them to the extreme with immaculately clean homes and healthy food are diagnosed with and succumb to cancer just like many young athletes in their prime.

The full spectrum of environmental pollution is in all likelihood the major cause of cancer and far more so than unhealthy lifestyles. If mentioned at all, the carcinogens encountered in our daily life are barely taken into account.

That flies right in the face of the research that identified carcinogens in industrial products such as building materials, paints, carpets, textile dyes in clothing, and chemicals in the soil, air, and water. Traces of herbicides, fungicides, pesticides, and insecticides used in agriculture as well as the hormones and steroids to raise livestock are found in our food. Potable water is tainted with detergents, nanoparticles, hormones, multi-resistant gram-negative bacteria, and chemical compounds used in polishes, paints, and the coatings perfluoroalkyl and polyfluoroalkyl (PFAS) that can't be filtered out in water treatment plants. The air is severely polluted with dioxides of carbon, nitrogen, and sulphur from industrial and vehicle emissions.

All of the above cause cancer!

Planet Earth is engulfed by carcinogens and more and more people suffer cancer thanks to mankind's unrelenting drive to systematically destroy or at least pollute what we need most to live and survive: clean air, water, soil, and an intact, healthy nature.

The more one digs, the more dirt one finds about those corporations that cause the problems and are protected by financial interests.

An investigative journalist uncovering this complexity will be condemned and chastised and in the worst case labelled 'anarchist' who has a beef with our way of life.

Thus, hardly anyone dares to touch this complex subject and the media relies on the hyped press releases of multi-billion dollar profit corporations of the manufacturing industry, the service sector of transport, tourism and junk food as well as chemical and pharmaceutical giants who all claim that their products and services are safe and a boon to humanity.

Cancer and the 'Health Service Industry'

The vast majority of medics and even more so the bureaucratic authorities of the 'Health Service Industry' appear to pay scant attention to scientifically-proven results of cancer treatment when they are achieved outside their respective turf.

Most medical practitioners will insist on the practice of "tried and true" methods they were taught in medical schools. They insist that the conventional treatment of cut, burn and poison is the only effective method of tackling cancer and propagate the bombastic claims of Big Pharma whose overpriced anticancer therapies treat cancer patients only in very rare cases with any kind of success.

It is noteworthy that the words 'heal' or 'cure' in conjunction with conventional anticancer therapies is never used. Usually a therapy is circumscribed with such militarist terms as 'attack', 'battle', 'kill' and 'war', which in reality has very little to do with the complicated task of understanding the origin and incessant growth of cancer cells and how to deal with the disease.

It leads one to conclude that the 'Health Service Industry' is overdue for a major revamp in its function and service to the public. It could be kick-started by governments legislating laws that oblige the pharma industry to provide actual proof of the alleged efficacy of its anticancer therapies and the benefits a cancer patient is supposed to derive from these medications.

That was the case in 2019 when the government of Italy passed laws to that effect. Others could follow this example but are too afraid of the wrath of Big Pharma whose annual profits from the sale of cancer medication alone exceed the gross domestic product (GDP) of many small countries.

At present the pharma companies' chemotherapies cause the cancer patients immense suffering and pain. Most of the therapies do not affect the cancer tumours sufficiently, if at all but will definitely attack and damage healthy cells. Therefore, health care experts who suggest a long-term benefit assessment of anticancer medications after their approval should get all the support they need from their respective governments. Any claimed efficacy of medications should be monitored for at least three years on the scale of administering them to patients who are supposed to benefit from it in the form of being cured of their illness at best or at least to experience a significant life extension and improvement of their quality of life.

Should a medication turn out to be useless or have a negative impact, the manufacturer should not only have to reimburse all consumers of that medication in full but also face penalties to compensate the patients and their families for their suffering.

That would be a first measure millions of people around the globe would welcome and show that the members of the legislative body of governments actually care about the health and welfare of their respective public with more than just words and empty phrases.

It would also make pharma companies more cautious about their claims of the efficacy of their medication and put a dent into their multi-billion-dollar annual profits gained from the sale of useless anticancer medication.

All the rest of the required 'Health Service Industry' reforms, ranging from weeding out bumptious, immoral medics to the streamlining of bureaucratic licensing procedures for medical professionals has to be left to the professional medical associations. They know what reforms are needed most urgently. It is just a question of them mustering the will and courage to do it.

Same Old, Same Old...

Big Pharma has no interest in funding trials that would be detrimental to its profit maximisation. The pharma industry insists on the maximum tolerated application of its drugs to the level of as much as a patient's body can take despite ample proof of the painful and often deadly side effects.

The tendency to recommend and wanting to prescribe costly anticancer therapies of which only a few under the best of circumstances have shown to prolong life or at least offer a better quality of life for the time of survival, is encountered around the world.

In case there is any doubt about the ineffectiveness of overpriced medication to cure a patient of cancer, the report of the World Cancer Day 2019[66] does support the argument.

The report stated that personalised medicine is the latest catchphrase that raises expectations and above all hopes. The pharmaceutical industry promises tailor-made therapies for the patient, highly effective, with few side effects and huge profits for the manufacturer in the area of cancer medicine. But personalised medicine also raises false expectations. It is not aimed at an individual patient, but at a group of people who share certain characteristics, which influence how medicines or therapies work.

Quote: "This is a billion-dollar business for the pharmaceutical industry. By tailoring a drug to an ever-smaller group of patients, they can accelerate the approval of an active ingredient and circumvent price regulations. Only years later, it will become clear whether the new drug really works and keeps its promise. Until then, the manufacturer has made oodles of money - at the expense of the hopes of the patient and his or her relatives."

---

[66] Ist medizinischer Fortschritt für alle bezahlbar?
Peter Mücke, NDR, 12th Sep. 2019
(https://www.tagesschau.de/inland/welt-krebs-tag-101.html)

What I stated before is confirmed when it says that "these cancer therapies cost €100,000 (US$120,000) and more a year for a single patient. Most of these drugs do not even promise a cure, but only an extension of life by a few weeks and months on average with a very questionable quality of life."

These enormous costs that the health care systems will inevitably have to deal with raises the question of how much they are willing to pay for the prolongation of the life of a patient. Some countries have already answered that question. In Britain, for example, a mathematical formula is used to stick a price tag on life extension. The National Healthcare System (NHS) only pays when the price of the therapy does not exceed a certain amount. It is time to discuss this uncomfortable topic in other countries, also and precisely so that in the end it doesn't come to such a bureaucratic and brutal solution, as is the case in Britain.

Cancer has no national boundaries. A cure achieved in a foreign country that is denied, prohibited, or too costly in your country may mean that you have to go to another one to get the help you need. Many American cancer sufferers can vouch for that being the only alternative. They go to Cuba[67] where they get effective medication at an affordable price that keeps their cancer in check.

In most instances it is not a case of these patients having eradicated their cancer with the medication they obtained in Cuba and decided to take. They still have cancer but stopped its life-threatening growth and spread and contained it. And managing the containment of cancer is a step towards the end of suffering that painful disease.

---

[67] Facing bleak odds, cancer patients chase one last chance - in Cuba
Rob Waters, 5th Aug. 2016
(https://www.statnews.com/2016/08/05/lung-cancer-cuba-biotech/)

The Future of Cancer Treatment

It is an ethical imperative that every doctor and patient understands the difference between absolute and relative risks to protect patients against unnecessary anxiety and manipulation.

Gerd Gigerenzer
Director, Harding Centre for Risk Literacy
Max Planck Institute for Human Development
Berlin, Germany

Innumerable scientists in the field of biopharmaceutical protein research and related areas such as immunology and molecular biology are exploring new methods and treatments to prevent, contain, and eradicate cancer. With a bit of fortitude and a lot of perseverance they will achieve that goal in the not too distant future.

However, it has to be stated clearly and succinctly that the "not too distant future" should be viewed in the context of research and development over the past fifty or sixty years. The progress of understanding the origins and spread of cancer that resulted in new therapies and treatments was slow for many years but has accelerated considerably since the early 2000s. Still, the major breakthrough that will ring in the end of this scourge should not be anticipated for a number of years.

Yet, the recent success of eradicating tumours and cancer cells with immunotherapy, albeit still on a limited scale but without surgical intervention, toxic drugs, and radiation treatment provides more than just a small ray of hope for the development of an effective treatment for a patient who has been diagnosed with cancer.

Also, the approach to containing the spread and growth of cancer tumours has achieved remarkable progress. Sadly, it appears to be limited to countries such as Cuba where leading oncologists are of the opinion that cancer cannot be totally eradicated but can be contained so that cancer patients live with the disease without suffering its severe, painful, and deadly consequences. Eventually and not just for medical but even more so for political reasons, the Cuban approach to cancer containment will overcome the hurdle of being recognised globally as the method that can help millions of people to live a productive and enjoyable life despite being afflicted with cancer.

The research and development of a vaccine that not only provides a cure for but also prevents cancer has been going on for about a decade. As was to be expected this huge task is a slow process since it does not just aim at one particular type of cancer but an effective treatment for cancer in general. Vaccines for five types of cancer are undergoing Phase I clinical trials at the time of this writing. It is anticipated that the researchers will be able to draw conclusions about similarities of the effect of the different vaccines in order to develop a broad-spectrum vaccine applicable to more than just five and hopefully all types of cancer. Since this undertaking is so complex in all its facets, it should not be expected to be crowned with success in the very near future but possibly in a timespan like a decade. Yet, in view of the development of cancer treatment since it began, one decade is equivalent to the not too distant future.

So, that is where we stand today - on the brink of great achievements in immunotherapy. In the meantime, bridging the gap between present and future treatments and therapies is necessary. It includes healthy food diets that strengthen the immune system as well as adjunct and adjuvant medications and unconventional methods that make conventional chemotherapy treatments effective to some degree.

You Are What You Eat

The food proffered to the masses of Americans and denizens of other countries for instant and constant consumption has been widely criticised and blasted with a range of expletives for causing obesity, cancer, and many other ailments.

A team from the Université Sorbonne Paris Cité, France, surveyed what people are eating.[68] The participants of the study were observed on average for five years. The result showed that an increase of ten percent in the proportion of ultra-processed food in the diet increases the number of cancer diagnoses by twelve percent.

Ultra-processed food was defined as including mass-produced bread and buns, sweet or savoury snacks including potato crisps, chocolate bars and sweets, soda pop and sweetened drinks, meatballs, poultry and fish nuggets, instant noodles and soups, frozen and ready meals, and treats made mostly or entirely from sugar, oils and fats.

Prof. Linda Bauld, Cancer Research UK's prevention expert, said: "It's already known that eating a lot of these foods can lead to weight gain, and being overweight or obese can also increase your risk of cancer. So, it's hard to disentangle the effects of diet and weight."

Most of the ultra-processed convenience foods are often identified as causing cancer or containing chemicals that are known to be carcinogenic. It is the poisonous cherry on top of the obesity causing foods.

A unique approach has been taken by a number of researchers who pursue the idea of specific diets that are supposed to prevent or even eradicate cancer.

Their ideas are based on the rediscovery of the research of the winner of the Nobel Prize for Medicine in 1923, the

---

[68] Ultra-processed foods 'linked to cancer'
James Gallagher, Health correspondent, 15th Feb. 2018
(http://www.bbc.com/news/health-43064290)

German physiologist Otto Warburg[69] who discovered "the nature and mode of action of the respiratory enzyme". He hypothesised that the root cause of cancer is oxygen deficiency, which creates an acidic state in the human body. Cancer cells are anaerobic and cannot survive in the presence of high levels of oxygen. He stated, "The prime cause of cancer is the replacement of the respiration of oxygen in normal body cells by a fermentation of sugar."

Based on Dr. Warburg's discoveries the research of diets aims to increase the oxygen in the blood stream to a level lethal to cancer or by preventing angiogenesis, the tumours' ability to develop new blood vessels that deliver nutrients.

This latter approach of promoting anti-angiogenesis has been pursued by Dr. William Li[70] whose suggested diet is beneficial for overall health and without a doubt much better than anti-angiogenic medications that have terrible side effects and can cause a patient's death. Dr. Li explains that a variety of foods, natural beverages, and herbs are laced with naturally occurring inhibitors of angiogenesis that starve cancer of nutrients. A 2011 study, published in the *Journal of Oncology*, showed the value of his anti-angiogenic diet to *prevent* cancer. Nobody can argue with that statement but if Dr. Li's diet is the non-plus-ultra of eradicating cancer tumours, as he claims, is still a matter of debate.

Another diet that has been widely criticised and put into the corner of quackery by staunch defenders of the cut, burn & poison doctrine is the ketogenic diet researched by Dominic D'Agostino[71] and Thomas Seyfried[72]. It is high in fat up from

[69] Dr. Otto Warburg, Biochemist and Physiologist, awarded the 1931 Nobel Prize for Medicine for his research on cellular respiration.
[70] Dr. William Li, physicist, founder and medical director of the Angiogenesis Foundation.
[71] Dominic D'Agostino, PhD, Associate Professor at the College of Medicine, University of South Florida.
[72] Dr. Thomas Seyfried, Professor of Biology at Boston College, Lead Researcher of the mechanisms of the ketogenic diet.

25% to 75%, protein up from 10% to 23%, and down in carbohydrates from 65% to 2%. It forces the body to burn fat rather than carbohydrates. The liver converts the fat into ketone bodies[73] that replace glucose as an energy source. The process of ketone supplementation and random fasting puts intense metabolic stress on cancer tumours that depend on glucose for their activity. D'Agostino and Seyfried state that the effects are a reduction in blood glucose and the mobilisation of fatty acids that starve tumours and suppress cancer growth. They rely on the discovery of Warburg that the primary difference between cancer cells and normal cells lies in the metabolic processes of using fermentation in place of respiration to create energy from nutrients. The evidence of preclinical and clinical studies of ketogenic diets in cancer therapy is limited and only provides weak evidence of anti-tumour effects with glioma and none in other cancers. Still, research continues and until conclusive evidence one way or the other is found, it should not be discarded as quackery. Potentially the diet could turn out to be useful as an adjunct to other therapies since one of the benefits is weightloss.

A healthy immune system is the first and possibly last line of defence against cancer. It is particularly important for older people to maintain a healthy diet to strengthen the immune system. There isn't strictly one food that can work wonders. So, it is crucial to have a balanced intake of a range of nutrients and avoid or at least reduce the ingestion of anything that weakens your immune system such as too much salt, too many calories, and alcohol.

A healthy diet would first of all include fibre. "If your gut bacteria isn't getting enough fibre to produce short-chain fatty acids, the immune cells won't function at their best," explains

---

[73] Ketone bodies - three related compounds (acetone, acetoacetic acid, beta-hydroxybutyric acid) produced during the metabolism of fats. *(Oxford Dictionary)*

Alex Ruani[74]. Good sources of fibre are whole grains (oat, rye, and brown rice), root vegetables (carrots and squash), raw fruit (apples, pears, and bananas), and legumes (red beans and lentils).

Amino acids assure the proper functioning of the immune system. Fish, chicken, eggs, yogurt, and cottage cheese provide all eight essential amino acids. Vegetarians and vegans should combine a variety of leafy greens, legumes, root vegetables, and grains for their intake of proteins that are made up of amino acids.

Fish is the source of omega 3 fatty acids that increase the immune response and are antioxidant and anti-inflammatory. However, caution is advised not to eat any fish like farmed Salmon, Cod, or Tilapia. They have been found to be chock full of antibiotics, pesticides, and flame-retardants in a study at the University of Albany, New York. Neither should you eat fish such as Shark, Swordfish, Marlin, Tuna, Perch, Halibut, Eel, and Sea Bass. They contain high levels of mercury and dioxin. Recommended are Snapper, Monk Fish, Anchovy, Flounder, Haddock, Herring, Sardine, Pilchard, Trout, Wild Salmon, and Mussels. They are all very high in omega 3 fatty acids and free of pathogens. The alternative for vegetarians and vegans are flaxseed, walnut, chia seed, shelled hemp seed, and sunflower seed.

Next on the list are vitamins. But the supplementary forms of pills are not recommended or necessary. They only cause you to produce very expensive urine that will ultimately pollute rivers and lakes. It is much better to stick to natural nutrients contained in regular fresh food.

Vitamin A promotes the function of T-cells and generates an antibody response. It is contained in beef and calf liver,

---

[74] Alex Ruani, Doctoral Researcher in Nutrition Science Education at University College London, and Chief Science Educator at The Health Sciences Academy
(https://thehealthsciencesacademy.org/thsa-alex-ruani/)

milk, cheese, yoghurt, carrots, cabbage, squash, pumpkin, melons, mangoes, tomatoes, broccoli, apricots, papayas, and tangerines. That's something for everybody.

Vitamin B6 raises the function of your immune system and the production of new immune cells. Another long list suggests noshing on wild salmon, turkey, red beans, cauliflower, bell peppers, bananas, squash, broccoli, asparagus, Brussels sprouts, lentils, and eggs.

Vitamin C became famous as the antidote to scurvy, which particularly affected poorly nourished sailors until the end of the 18th century. Now it is known to support also anti-microbial and NK-cell functions and increases the blood levels of antibodies. It is contained at high levels in cabbage, broccoli, spinach, peas, cauliflower, strawberries, kiwis, melons, tomatoes, and all citrus fruits.

Vitamin D has been found in recent studies to slow or prevent the development of cancer, decrease cancer cell growth, stimulate cancer cell death, and reduce tumour blood vessel formation. It is sometimes called the "sunshine vitamin" because it is produced in your skin in response to sunlight. If you can, catch a few rays of sunshine for fifteen minutes a day. More isn't necessary for all the Vitamin D you need. And on a rainy day or in the darkness of winter you can rely on the food under the A, B, and C vitamins.

And finally, the list of essentials of a healthy diet has to include iron, zinc, flavonoids [75], and probiotics [76]. These elements support a rapid response of the immune system to a pathogen, immune cell proliferation, antibacterial activity, enzyme function, and improve dendritic cell and T-cell functions. The list appears almost endless with pork, pumpkin

---

[75] Flavonoid - a biologically active compound found in plants.

[76] Probiotic - a substance, which stimulates the growth of microorganisms, especially those with beneficial properties such as those of the intestinal flora.

seeds, almonds, cashew nuts, Brazil nuts, pecans, sesame seeds, walnuts, dates, or raisins as a source for iron, lamb, haddock, egg yolks, ginger root, dried split peas, green peas, turnips, whole wheat grain, rye, oats, and peanuts for your supply of zinc, green or black tea, citrus fruit, berries, spinach, apples, cacao for flavonoids, and last but not least yoghurt, soft cheese, tempeh, kefir, sauerkraut, miso, and kimchi as a source of probiotics.

So, you see, it should be easy to maintain a healthy diet that helps to strengthen your immune system. Most of the listed foods are plentiful and many are very affordable as well. All you have to do is stay away from processed food and apply a bit of elbow grease making a delicious meal from scratch with your favourite ingredients. Just let your culinary imagination run wild and start to live healthy.

Ignored Orphan Medications

Continuous advances in medical R&D will eventually replace the "tried and true" conventional methods and put them on the garbage dump of medical history like the treatment of cancer with mustard gas that was still practised widely in the 1950s. However, the stranglehold of bureaucracy and Big Pharma over the medical profession has to be broken first.

When the curative effect of a medication has been proven in various trials and its practical application, medical practitioners should not be hindered by the health ministries' and other official bodies' paternalism that is underlying medical practice to prescribe and administer the drug even on an experimental basis to save a patient's life.

In order to forestall further speculations and criticism concerning the prescription of so-called orphan medications for cancer patients, their antitumor effect needs to be investigated in empirical clinical trials with respect to metabolism and tolerability of each drug and often in combination with approved, standard chemotherapeutic agents. And that poses a huge problem.

A clinical trial usually requires at least two hundred and preferably several thousand cancer patients to participate, especially patients that are beyond conventional therapy.

One half of the group, whose standard anticancer medication hasn't had any beneficial effect, have the trial medication not only administered as an adjunct to help anticancer medication to be effective, but also as an adjuvant, a substance that enhances the patient's immune system to respond to an antigen and is given after other therapies have failed to achieve a desired result. The other half of the group of patients is given a placebo, e.g. a sugar pill. It means that patients beyond therapy that are given a placebo will die.

The Health Industry insists on such clinical trials to provide what is in their opinion 'proof absolute' of the efficacy of a medication. Problem is that there are few if any doctors willing to watch several hundred cancer patients die in sheer agony while the other half of the test-group potentially survives, is free of pain, and walks out of the hospital after a curative treatment of their cancer.

Such procedure is medieval and one has to question why positive results achieved in a controlled clinical trial cannot be accepted as proof of a medication's efficacy. When positive results with an extensive test group of patients have been achieved, the medication should be noted as effective and made available commercially.

Besides the technologies, techniques, treatment methods, R&D of proteins that hold promise in the advancement of immunotherapy there are adjunct and adjuvant orphan medications that may not relate directly to immunotherapy but do improve conventional therapies to a vast extent.

Missing in Action, as Jake Bernstein[77] puts it, are these low-cost orphan medications - therapies or medications created to treat cancer, including generics that are investigated for their anticancer effect - that don't have enough profit potential for pharma companies to invest in researching them.

As is the case with medications in other fields of application, for example malaria vaccine and antibiotics[78], when pharma companies can't make whopping profits, they are not interested in producing the medicine.

In another report titled "How Big Pharma Holds Back in the War on Cancer",[79] Bernstein addresses and documents

---

[77] MIA In The War On Cancer: Where Are The Low-Cost Treatments? *Jake Bernstein, ProPublica, 23rd April 2014 (https://www.propublica.org/article/where-are-the-low-cost-cancer-treatments)*

[78] Big Pharma nixes new drugs despite impending 'antibiotic apocalypse' *(https://www.dw.com/en/big-pharma-nixes-new-drugs-despite-impending-antibiotic-apocalypse/a-50432213)*

[79] How Big Pharma Holds Back in the War on Cancer *Jake Bernstein, ProPublica, 12th July 2017*

how the research of affordable and effective cancer medications is suppressed by Big Pharma on a global scale and, worse yet, how this research and development mostly does not receive support, financially or otherwise, from the respective governments of the countries where it is conducted. Rarely do generic orphan medications receive funding for clinical trials to prove the efficacy in cancer treatment. Normally, Big Pharma provides funding for elaborate and lengthy trials. Naturally, it will oppose the discovery of any medication that may toss more than a handful of gravel into its flogging of overpriced chemotherapies to millions of cancer patients who fall for the unsubstantiated claims of life extension and a better quality of life.

Actually, Big Pharma is extremely active in trying to stop all research of affordable and effective cancer medications on a global scale and persuading the respective governments to prevent any kind of support for what they consider to be 'nefarious and counterproductive' activities. They go as far as threatening to withdraw all research and development activities from countries that do not abide by their demand although they do hardly any R&D, which is done in the laboratories of universities and financed with tax dollars.

A telling example to this effect is provided by Michelle Holmes[80]. She has been trying for years to raise money for trials of the effects of Aspirin on breast cancer. Animal studies, *in vitro* experiments, and the analysis of patient outcomes suggest that Aspirin might help inhibit breast cancer from spreading. Yet even her peers on scientific advisory boards appear uninterested. She says, "A drug that could be patented would get a randomised trial, but Aspirin, which has amazing properties, goes unexplored because it's 99 cents at

---

[80] Michelle Holmes, Associate Professor, Department of Epidemiology, Brigham and Women's Hospital, Channing Lab
Aspirin intake and survival after breast cancer. J Clin Oncology, 2010 Mar 20;28(9):1467-72. (PMC 2849768)

the local drugstore," and adds, "What is scientific and sexy is driven by what can be monetised and that becomes the norm."

Another example of the lack of financial support is a small retrospective study of 327 mastectomy patients, conducted by Patrice Forget[81], University Hospital Brussels. The anti-inflammatory non-toxic generic drug Ketorolac[82] has shown to prevent the post-operative recurrence and metastasis of breast cancer. Ketorolac is administered just before or after a surgical intervention. Should the study confirm its efficacy then it would have to undergo a randomised clinical trial with thousands of patients around the world. So far there has been little indication that the required funding for such a trial has been or can be raised.

This is tragic to say the least because the evidence collected to date shows that administering Ketorolac could save thousands of lives. [83] Approximately 30% of all women afflicted with breast cancer or well over 600,000 still die every year as a result of its recurrence and metastasis. Ketorolac could help to prevent this and should get the financial support it needs for an empirical clinical trial.

Researchers at Harvard University and other leading institutions have come to the conclusion that Ketorolac may be an effective treatment for other forms of cancer as well. But since administering this generic drug costs as little as $1 (one dollar) per application, it has been proven difficult to raise the required funding for any further investigation.

---

[81] Prof. Patrice Forget, M.D. Ph.D., Clinical Professor in Anaesthesia and Pain Medicine, Belgium, and President, Belgian Pain Society.
(https://www.abdn.ac.uk/iahs/research/epidemiology/ profiles/ patrice.forget)

[82] Ketorolac, brand name Toradol among others, is a nonsteroidal anti-inflammatory drug (NSAID) used to treat pain.
(en.wikipedia.org/wiki/Ketorolac)

[83] Is this One Dollar Pill a Breast Cancer Breakthrough?
Ralph Moss, PhD, 28th Dec. 2018
(https://www.mossreports.com/breast-cancer-pill-ketorolac/)

Michael Retsky and Romano Demicheli wrote a book[84] about the benefits of administering Ketorolac and suggest that every woman who undergoes breast cancer surgery should take it within the recommended dosage framework. Also, they agree with Patrice Forget that the investigation of this drug should be expanded to other types of cancer.

---

[84] Perioperative Inflammation as Triggering Mechanism of Metastasis Development, *Michael W. Retsky, Romano Demicheli Springer-Nature Book, ISBN-13: 978-3319579429*

Could D,L-Methadone be the Answer?

Another prominent example of an orphan medication that had been denied a clinical trial until 2019 is D,L-methadone. But before the trials and tribulations of methadone are explained, it should be noted that methadone is listed by the WHO *'Essential Medicines'* as a safe and effective medicine required in any health care system. It is a globally approved analgesic, which sheds a strange light on oncologists and palliative cares specialists who adamantly refuse to prescribe and administer it.

When D,L-methadone research results were published that provided proof of its efficacy as a cancer adjunct, the medical community was suddenly in what can only be described as panic. The publication of Dr. Friesen's report as well as its broadcast on ABC News[85] in North America in August 2008 caused uproar.

Although research, retrospective and prospective trials as well as the "off-label" treatment of more than 5,000 cancer patients over a period of twenty years provided proof of its efficacy as an adjunct and adjuvant medication, the German Cancer Society had been 'persuaded' not to finance the clinical trial it had demanded for over ten years.

It took a public outcry and intervention of prominent cancer specialists until German Cancer Aid provided funding of €1.6 million (US$1.75 million) for a clinical trial of one type of cancer.

That amounts to a stinging backhander for the scientists who researched and discovered the medication's efficacy because the funding is tied to the demand of having to provide proof of a curative effect of D,L-methadone for a total of 12 types of cancer before it can be authorised and licensed as a publicly available adjunct medication.

---

[85] Methadone Kills Resistant Leukemia Cells, *1ˢᵗ Aug. 2008,*
  (http://abcnews.go.com/Health/Healthday/story?id=5499629)

Is that going to be another victory for Big Pharma? It will do everything in its power to prevent this medicine from entering the market as a licensed anti-cancer medication. Already some oncologists are asking the obvious question: How can a medicine that costs about €85 (US$92) for one year of effective treatment be better than a medication that costs over €100,000 (US$120,000)?

With any luck and a lot of persistence it is going to be a victory for the proponents of D,L-methadone because more and more medical practitioners help their cancer patients with the "off-label" prescription and see them thrive and lead a normal life as explained in the following narrative.

An oncologist[86] describes to a patient who had suffered Stage IV Glioblastoma how D,L-methadone helped to cure him of his brain cancer and return to a productive life.

"Every tumour has opioid receptors. D,L-methadone is able to dock onto these cells due to its molecular structure. As a result, the surface of a tumour cell is damaged, which provides access for the patient's immune system cells as well as reduced amounts of the chemo substances that are used to treat cancer to enter the tumour.

"Tumour cells begin to pump out the chemotherapeutic agents and immune cells after a certain time and become resistant. This process is prevented by D,L-methadone when drug and immune cells stay in the cancer cell in higher concentrations than before and kill the cell from the inside.

"It should be noted that the methadone for substitution therapy is laevorotatory or L-methadone by itself and in its function quite different from the racemic D,L-methadone.

"L-methadone is a micron-opioid receptor agonist that initiates a physiological response when combined with a receptor and a higher intrinsic activity than morphine but a

---

[86] Methadone Therapy Medically Explained by Dr. med. Dietmar Peikert (*https://www.youtube.com/watch?v=wbHwktofm2w*)

lower degree to which it tends to combine with opioid receptors. D-methadone does not affect opioid receptors but binds to the receptors related to glutamate and thus assists the L-methadone to cling to the cancer cell receptors. It acts as a receptor antagonist against glutamate.

"Thus, the dextrorotatory and laevorotatory action of the racemic D,L-methadone activates the opioid receptors located on the surface of the cancer cells. Opening the receptors by damaging the surface of cancer cells is achieved due to multiple receptor affinities. D,L-methadone clings to the receptors of cancer cells and tumours, breaks down their surface structure, and opens them for the penetration by lymphocytes and medication.

"This function was noted by the palliative care specialist Hilscher when he replaced the morphine preparations for the patients in his hospice with D,L-methadone. Many terminally ill cancer patients recovered, were cured, and became healthy. He investigated the phenomenon and contacted various universities with a request for research.

"The biologist Claudia Friesen [87] of the Biochemical Research Institute, University of Ulm, discovered the effect of the drug. She had investigated cancer tumours and found that each one has opioid receptors. Her experiment of exposing leukaemia cells to D,L-methadone resulted in the death of the cancer cells. Ironically, she put that result down to her experiment having gone wrong. It had not been the aim of her research. She replicated the result many times before she finally realised that she had discovered something astounding.

"Dr. Friesen and Dr. Hilscher developed the formulation of D,L-methadone that is not life threatening. The only negative side effects of ingesting D,L-methadone at the prescribed dosage are constipation and nausea in the first four weeks for

---

[87] Methadone, *Dr. Claudia Friesen, University Hospital Ulm (https://www.gesundheitsindustriebw.de/en/article/news/methadone-the-last-step-to-becoming-an-anti-cancer-drug/)*

opioid naïve patients. The positive side effect is its mood and appetite enhancing outcome."

Following her discovery and development of the aqueous solution, Dr. Friesen researched the effect for 10 years. Her findings: D,L-methadone has a major impact on all types of cancer cells. Also liver and lung metastases declined, the symptoms of the disease disappeared, and the cancer cells were killed.[88] Her research papers were published after peer review in the following scientific publications:

- *Journal of the American Association for Cancer Research*[89]
- *RxPG News - Peer Reviewed News for Medical Professionals, USA*[90]
- *Anticancer Research - International Journal of Cancer Research and Treatment, USA*[91]

Further support for D,L-methadone came from a team of microbiologists and urologists who researched it for a number of years. They state that methadone has beneficial characteristics as an analgesic, high bioavailability, and multiple receptor affinities. The advantage of D,L-methadone is that is has no active metabolites, which could interfere with

---

[88] Methadone, Commonly Used as Maintenance Medication for Outpatient Treatment of Opioid Dependence, Kills Leukemia Cells and Overcomes Chemoresistance
Claudia Friesen, Mareike Roscher, Andreas Alt and Erich Miltner (https://cancerres.aacrjournals.org/content/68/15/6059)

[89] Methadone, Commonly Used as Maintenance Medication for Outpatient Treatment of Opioid Dependence, Kills Leukemia Cells, and Overcomes Chemoresistance, *August 2008*
Claudia Friesen, Mareike Roscher, Andreas Alt and Erich Miltner, (https://cancerres.aacrjournals.org/content/68/15/6059.long)

[90] Methadone - promising treatment for cancer, *2nd Aug. 2008*
(http://www.rxpgnews.com/cancer-research/Methadone - promising_treatment_for_cancer_printer.shtml)

[91] Safety and Tolerance of D,L-Methadone in Combination with Chemotherapy in Patients with Glioma, *March 2017*
Julia Onken, Claudia Friesen, Peter Vajkoczy, and Martin Misch (http://ar.iiarjournals.org/content/37/3/1227.long#ref-list-1)

kidney and liver function. Evidence of their preclinical studies showed that methadone elicits antitumor activity by downregulating the threshold of apoptosis and enhancing the effects of different chemotherapeutic agents. Various preclinical studies had demonstrated that methadone also acts as an enhancer of apoptosis in cancer cells of different origin.[92]

At the 2016 Symposium on Pain and Palliative Care in Frankfurt/Main, Germany, the palliative care specialist Dr. Hilscher said, "D,L-methadone induces a physiological apoptosis, the growth of tumours is inhibited, but it alone does not cure cancer. When we combine D,L-methadone with cytotoxic drugs, we see great results."

The aqueous solution is effective with all solid tumours and glioblastomas according to his experience. Yet, patients with glioblastomas who receive this therapy often die as a result of radiogenic dementia. "It is very bitter to see patients, who no longer have brain tumours, die from the side effects of radiotherapy," said Hilscher.[93]

Dr. Friesen collected the data of more than 350 cancer patients, most of them bedridden. When they started to take D,L-methadone, they could lead a normal life and often valued the improvement of their quality of life alone sufficient for using the medication. All of the patients' magnetic resonance imaging (MRI) showed a marked decrease in metastases and all tumours showed positive progression towards being destroyed.

Proof of the aqueous solution D,L-methadone's efficacy and benefits in pain management for cancer patients was

---

[92] Methadone as a "Tumor Theralgesic" against Cancer
Marta Michalska et al, University Freiburg, Germany, October 2017 (https://www.researchgate.net/publication/320732103_Methadone_as_a_Tumor_Theralgesic_against_Cancer)
[93] Methadone: A misunderstood analgesic - with anti-tumor effects
(http://deutsch.medscape.com/artikelansicht/4904685)

established over two decades ago as a result of multi-year studies in Europe, Australia, and Canada[94]. It is prescribed in Europe and Australia, however rarely, for outpatient titration in the treatment of cancer pain.

The various trials and results of the practical application documented instant pain relief, prolongation of life, and the apoptosis of cancer cells. All of it was dismissed.[95] What was the underlying reason? It is too cheap! And that poses a major problem when a clinical trial proves that such medication has a curative effect.

There is no pharma company in the world willing to produce a medication as a commercial product that is too cheap because profits would be absolutely minimal! Big Pharma has not come forward expressing interest in the production of cheap anti-cancer medications specifically because there is relatively little money to be made, not the billions that shareholders would expect despite millions of potential customers.

Also, the benefits of the racemic mix D,L-methadone are not acknowledged by many health authorities, professional medical associations, and the vast majority of medical practitioners. The compound is simply tossed into the mix of deadly opioids and recommended only for substitution therapy and the detoxification of drug addicts. It is incomprehensible that oncologists, palliative care specialists as well as professional medical associations do not differentiate between preparations of L-methadone for drug replacement therapy and the standard recipe aqueous solution

---

[94] Methadone: Outpatient Titration and Monitoring Strategies in Cancer Patients *Neil A. Hagen, MD, FRCPC, and Eric Wasylenko, MD Journal of Pain and Symptom Management, 5th Nov. 1999*

[95] Bei Methadon wird grundsätzlich alles infrage gestellt! *Dr. rer. nat. Claudia Friesen, 6th Nov. 2019 (https://www.coliquio.de/wissen/ Praxis-Wissen-kompakt-100/Claudia-Friesen-Bei-Methadon-wird-grundsaetzlich-alles-infrage-gestellt-100)*

161

racemic D,L-methadone for cancer patients. Their minds are so transfixed on methadone as an opioid substitute that they will not accept scientific proof or the evidence of medical records of thousands of patients who were treated successfully for cancer.

Commercial preparations for drug replacement therapy and detoxification contain a very high level of 250mg to 750mg of L-methadone administered orally, intravenously, or rectally up to four times a day. In contrast, the aqueous solution D,L-methadone contains 1g of the opioid in 100ml of purified water and is administered sublingually at a dosage of 0.25ml (2.5mg) to 1ml (10mg) only twice a day. L-methadone given to drug addicts would not be beneficial in the apoptosis of cancer cells and has been proven to be deadly for cancer patients.

Even the scientific evidence of the research documented in a report published in August 2008 could not persuade the medical community to give it favourable considerations[96]. Detractors dismissed the research results as anecdotal and charlatanry, i.e. that this German biomedical doctor who had discovered it was pushing a fake remedy. Yet, none of the detractors provided proof of having administered D,L-methadone at the recommended dosage and intervals to any of their patients.

A truly pathetic example was set by the director of the neurological clinic at Heidelberg University Hospital. He caused a sensation with a study of methadone in cancer therapy by treating brain tumour cells with L-methadone and chemotherapy. He concluded that methadone does not cause the death of cancer cells. Please note: He used L-methadone

---

[96] Methadone, Commonly Used as Maintenance Medication for Outpatient Treatment of Opioid Dependence, Kills Leukemia Cells, and Overcomes Chemoresistance, *August 2008*
Claudia Friesen, Mareike Roscher, Andreas Alt and Erich Miltner (https://cancerres.aacrjournals.org/content/68/15/6059.long)

that does not prevent the down-regulation of the opioid receptors on the tumour cell surface as it is the case with D,L-methadone. He did not work with cell cultures that had enough receptors for opioids, did not investigate the effect of D,L-methadone, and used a chemotherapeutic agent that only works after metabolism. He was severely criticised for his faulty study but being the director of a NeuroOncology Program, the result of his study was accepted. The criticism was ignored,[97] which is in line with the somewhat sarcastic phrase that one has to bow before titled people until one's arse has the highest rank.

Other doctors went as far as publishing horror stories about patients who had self-administered the drug without supervision and died within days. They forgot to mention that these patients had heard of the effect of methadone and in their despair had taken the medication normally given to drug addicts for drug replacement therapy at a dosage of more than one hundred times the proposed quantity for patients who are or have been undergoing cancer therapy.

In Germany not only individual doctors but also the German Cancer Society had warned of unspecified 'terrible' side effects of D,L-methadone. In a mixture of ignorance, propaganda, and economic interests it contributed to the bad reputation of the racemic preparation.

Furthermore, a lot of resistance will be encountered when a cancer patient asks a doctor to prescribe the "off label" medication. Instead, the patient will be warned about the dangers and the probability of addiction and death.

Think about that for a moment. It is ridiculous! A cancer patient at death's door who has become addicted to opioids due to the regular administration of morphine or fentanyl is

---

[97] Methadone in cancer therapy: the most important Q & A
Stefanie Schmidt / David Nau, 28th Dec. 2018
(https://www.swp.de/ suedwesten/staedte/ulm/methadon-in-der-krebstherapie-fragen-und-antworten-28025448.html)

warned that a minute amount of about one-hundredth of the heroin addiction substitute of a proven synthetic opioid causes addiction and death! It makes one want to yell at the doctor to wake up, realise that the patient is at death's door, the medication improves the quality of life, prolongs life, functions as a chemo-sensitiser, helps to kill cancer cells and, thus, can help to cure the patient!

Detractors of proven medical research results are a global problem. A team of doctors who declared methadone to be unproven and dangerous quite unintentionally gave the true reason for denouncing it. They stated that proof of a curative effect of D,L-methadone in treating cancer would result in the public's total loss of confidence in the drugs of the pharma industry. Yes! Absolutely!

A further denigration of the racemic aqueous solution was provided by the president of German Society for Palliative Medicine[98] who condemns the use of methadone in cancer therapy although his colleagues see it very differently. He claims that the use of methadone in cancer therapy is merely a matter of clutching at straws and then goes on to ridicule himself by stating that these straws are used only to do business. At €85 (US$92) for one year of effective treatment, I have to ask what business he had in mind. There is hardly a profit to be made in contrast to the billions Big Pharma rakes in with its overpriced medicines.

Final results of D,L-methadone's ongoing clinical trial are anticipated to be announced by the end of 2021. That is something eagerly awaited by millions of cancer patients.

---

[98] How Palliative Care Professionals rate methadone differently in cancer therapy, *Beatrice Hamberger, 28th June 2017* *(https://www.gesundheitsstadt-berlin.de/so-unterschiedlich-bewerten-palliativmediziner-methadon-in-der-krebstherapie-11490/)*

An Unconventional Cancer Therapy

Michael Retsky, who supports the investigation of Ketorolac, appears to be a bit of a maverick when it comes to investigating and supporting unconventional cancer therapies and treatments as well. [99] Originally a physicist he switched to cancer research some thirty years ago and has become a recognised authority in his field of activity at the Harvard School of Public Health, Boston. He was diagnosed with Stage III colon cancer in 1994 and rejected the conventional maximum tolerated chemotherapy after surgery. It was based on his research of tumour growth and therapy. Instead he relied on the metronomic chemotherapy developed by William Hrushesky, MD,[100] although it had never been used as an adjuvant therapy.

The metronomic chemotherapy was a low dose measured infusion of the colon cancer drug 5-fluorouracil (5FU) administered at night for 5 hours with a portable pump over a period of two years. It was anti-angiogenic, non-toxic, and worked very well as he proved with his treatment. He had no recurrence or metastasis and has been cancer-free since.

As it is the case with Aspirin and Ketorolac, the low dose metronomic infusion of cancer drugs also does not receive financial support for a large-scale investigation and empirical clinical trials with thousands of patients. Big Pharma insists on administering the conventional maximum tolerated chemotherapy although a low dose infusion could prove that at least some of its chemotherapies actually work and are beneficial to cancer patients.

---

[99] Michael W. Retsky, Ph.D., Research Associate, Harvard T.H. Chan School of Public Health
(https://connects.catalyst.harvard.edu/ Profiles/display/Person/1089)

[100] Dr. William Hrushesky, MD is a Medical Oncology Specialist in West Orange, NJ and has over 47 years of experience in the medical field.
(https://www.healthgrades.com/physician/dr-william-hrushesky-yrn48)

Thinking Outside the Box

Every oncologist knows that a cancer cell divides rapidly and out of control. It needs more and different building materials than a healthy cell. It also has a significantly higher number of receptors than a healthy cell. They are embedded in the cell's epidermis to receive the nutrients it needs to grow and function as a defence mechanism as well.

A cancer cell appears to recognise anything that might endanger its survival and shut itself off from being penetrated by anticancer medication. Its receptors pretend to be that of a healthy cell, which signals to the immune system not to attack it. A medication has to break through the cancer cell's defence for the body's immune system cells to penetrate and destroy the tumour. But what exactly is that evidently insurmountable defence system of cancer cells?

The Dutch researcher Lenneke Cornelissen[101] studied these defences of cancer tumours and detected a surprising coincidence. She started out by questioning why a healthy immune system kills bacteria and viruses but not a cancer tumour, in other words, what is the tumour's defence mechanism. Following the line of logic that a cancer cell growing in the body should be recognised as foreign to the system and should be killed, she considered an embryo or foetus that is genetically made up of cells from the mother and the father in relatively equal parts should therefore be recognised by the mother's immune system as a foreign body as well and should be treated as such. She knew that a glycan structure, a wall of compounds consisting of a large number of monosaccharides, basic units of carbohydrates, that is built around the embryo from its earliest stage, functions as a defensive shield against an attack from the pregnant woman's immune system.

---

[101] Lenneke Cornelissen, MSc, postdoc in OncoImmunology
Radboud University Medical Centre, Amsterdam, Netherlands.

166

Investigating cancer tumours, she found that the tumours from an early stage in their development build a glycan structure on the cell surface identical to the one built around a foetus to protect them against attacks from the immune system. That is the defence shield that renders the immune system in most instances ineffective in eliminating cancer cells[102] since it is not possible to penetrate the tumour.

She is researching cancer specific glycan structures to learn how the interaction between the immune system and these structures is blocked. The defensive shield has to be perforated or destroyed for the immune system to effectively enter and destroy a tumour.

Ms. Cornelissen is just one of the multitudes of young cancer researchers around the world who have dedicated themselves to finding answers to the pressing questions of what the best and most effective method is to eradicate cancer cells without doing harm to healthy tissue and cells. She follows the path of more and more scientists who do their research in the field of cancer immunotherapy that aims to enable the body's immune system to fulfil its function of eliminating not just bacteria and viruses but all pathogens that cause disease. Achieving that goal without subjecting a cancer patient to toxic medications is the challenge she and the medical community at large are facing.

Timo Betz[103], another researcher who thinks outside the box, questioned how the metastasis of cancer tumours functions. As a physicist/biologist he thought about the mechanics of cancer to find out how tumours spread the

---

[102] Bittersweet symphony: How tumor-associated glycan structures orchestrate immune evasion, *Lenneke Cornelissen* (*https://cancerimmunolres.aacrjournals.org/content/6/9_Supplement/B63*)

[103] Prof. Dr. Timo Betz, Physicist/Biologist, University of Münster, Germany (*The Mechanics of Cancer - TED^x*)

cancer cells and let them migrate in all directions at once. All aggressive forms of cancer share those migrating cells called metastasis.

He observed that the cancer cells do not loosely float around but have to attach to something to leave the tumour and move somewhere else. They use collagen, the main structural protein found in animal connective tissue to overcome the cell-cell adhesion of the tumour and move out simultaneously in all directions. The cancer cells migrate only when they can create the necessary tension in the collagen. Consequently, when this process of creating tension is interrupted by cutting the collagen, metastasis becomes impossible.

Hence he concluded with the following observations that should be taken into consideration to stop metastasis:

- metastasis is a mechanical event
- cancer cells will change their environment to facilitate and support metastasis
- cancer cells don't need a genetically encoded program to change their environment
- one should interfere with collagen to prevent metastasis instead of focusing on a tumour and targeting it.

His conclusions are significant since they are in line with the opinion of many cancer researchers that it is not the prime tumour that kills a patient but the metastasis.

His and Ms. Cornelissen's research are remarkable contributions in the field of cancer research and provide important facets to finding a cure that will eradicate cancer for good.

A Look at Immunotherapy

It has to be understood that cancer is not a freak aberration but a completely normal occurrence, in the words of Dr. Leonard Sender,[104] to appreciate new developments and the potential future of cancer treatment.

Cancer cells are developed all the time to the tune of billions of cells being regenerated in our bodies every day. Cell division, another normal process, can lead to a cancer cell. A well-functioning and highly active immune system detects these early cancer cells and destroys them. When a cancer cell escapes the surveillance of the immune system and starts its cell division, it develops over a time of many years, into the full-blown cancer of a tumour large enough to be detected during a screening process.

The development of cancer cells is with us all the time from cradle to grave, so to speak. It is a continuum and not a case of every human being having cancer several times in a life span. Furthermore, cancer is never acute, meaning that it doesn't pop up out of nowhere from one day to the next as full-blown cancer with golf-ball size tumours. It is a slow developmental process over months and years of a tiny healthy cell becoming cancerous, escaping the immune system, and eventually growing to a size that is large enough to be identified as a malignant tumour.

Consequently, it is extremely rare to detect cancer at Stage I or II when it could be eradicated with relative ease. When it is detected, it is usually due to secondary symptoms such as lumps, sores that fail to heal, abnormal bleeding, pain from persistent indigestion, or jaundice when cancer is already at Stage III or IV. Researchers have been pondering various approaches and different solutions in their search for methods or tools that allow for the early detection of cancer.

---

[104] Dr. Leonard S. Sender, MD
University of the Witwatersrand, Johannesburg, South Africa, Pediatric, Adolescent and Young Adult Oncology.

In this endeavour the team of Cancer Research UK in Cambridge[105] has come up with a project of collecting breath samples of some 1,500 participants to find out if a breath test could detect the presence of cancer at an early stage. If this technology yields the result it is intended to achieve, the breath test could be used alongside blood and urine samples to help general practitioners to detect signs of cancer and refer the patient for more detailed tests to cancer clinics. Among the participants are people that have been diagnosed with oesophageal and stomach cancers and will include people with prostate, kidney, bladder, liver, and pancreatic cancers as well as healthy people.

The test detects volatile organic compound molecules that are released by biochemical reactions of cells in the body. When cancer is present, the cells produce a different pattern of molecules and a different smell. Using breath biopsy this difference can be identified in the breath and the ultimate aim is to see if different types of cancer produce different patterns. In short, the team is not only aiming to detect cancer per se but also to identify various types of cancer.

The project was started in early 2019 and will take several years until conclusive results are obtained. Dr. David Crosby, head of early detection research at Cancer Research UK, said breath tests are a technology that has the potential "to revolutionise the way we detect and diagnose cancer in the future".

The Bioengineer Dr. Raj Krishnan[106] developed a system that facilitates a cancer diagnosis in fifteen minutes or less with the discovery of biomarkers measured in a blood sample

---

[105] Is a breath test key to detecting cancer?
BBC News, Health, 3rd Jan. 2019
(https://www.bbc.com/news/health-46746552)
[106] Raj Krishnan, Ph.D. in Bioengineering, UC SanDiego, revolutionary cancer diagnosis at its earliest stage with the discovery of biomarkers in blood samples.

that reflect early stage cancer. Such a speedy diagnosis in itself is a breakthrough and should be welcome.

Yet, this early stage speedy diagnosis stands in stark contrast to the results of a study published in the Medical Journal of Australia.[107] It established the lifetime risks of melanoma and lung, breast, prostate, renal, and thyroid cancers, the types with significant occurrence in Australia. The majority of these cancers diagnosed might reasonably be attributed to overdiagnosis by comparing the difference in current and past lifetime risks of cancer.

The Australian study was confirmed in the British Medical Journal[108] about "too much screening of asymptomatic individuals, too much investigation of those with symptoms, too much reliance on biomarkers, too many quasi-diseases, too much diagnosis often leading to too much treatment, sometimes cost-ineffective, administering medicines that are too costly and too rapidly approved for marketing, too many adverse reactions, and too much inappropriate monitoring."

And a report in Canada[109] warned, "Overdiagnosis means identifying problems that weren't causing symptoms and were never going to cause the patient harm" and continues, "Harm may come from cancer treatment of patients who would never have had symptoms in their lifetime."

It leads to the conclusion that an early stage cancer speedy diagnosis would only be truly useful if Raj Krishnan's system could differentiate between cancer cell mutations that will become full-blown cancer and the ones that can be safely ignored to avoid overdiagnosis and treatment when a healthy

---

[107] Estimating the magnitude of cancer over-diagnosis in Australia
(https://onlinelibrary.wiley.com/doi/full/10.5694/ mja2.50455)
[108] Over-diagnosis: what it is and what it isn't
(https://ebm.bmj.com/content/23/1/1)
[109] Why a growing number of cancers may best be left untreated
Dr. Brian Goldman
CBC News, 26th Jan. 2020

and fully functioning immune system takes care of the cancer cells as was suggested by the Pan-Cancer Analysis of Whole Genomes. Possibly this could be improved by expanding the function of the early stage cancer diagnosis system to include an assessment of the immune system status of a tested person.

As Dr. Sender said, "a well-functioning and highly active immune system detects ... early cancer cells and destroys them". It contraindicates Raj Krishnan's early stage cancer diagnosis system. Early stage cancer detection that does not test the immune system and determines if its health and strength could result in unnecessary anti-cancer treatment that will actually cause harm to healthy cells, organs, and tissue especially with conventional chemo- and radiotherapy.

Considering the damage done to healthy cells and tissue by chemo- and radiotherapy, a vast number of medical practitioners and scientists have turned to researching the immune system for a cure. Their aim is to get to know a cancer cell better and learn what makes the "enemy" tick. What are the inner workings of a cancer cell? What triggers the growth of a healthy cell into a cancer cell and life-threatening metastasis? What causes these cells to continue fighting a "foreign invader that is no longer there"?

Dr. Steven Rosenberg[110], chief of surgery at the National Cancer Institute, Baltimore, Maryland, USA, one of the world's leading centres of cancer research, pioneered the development of effective immunotherapies and gene therapies for patients with advanced cancers.

He has had remarkable success with a so-called 'living drug' made from a patient's own cells.[111] He stated that it is

---

[110] Steven A. Rosenberg, M.D., Ph.D., Chief, Surgery Branch, Senior Investigator, Head, Tumor Immunology Section, National Cancer Institute, Centre for Cancer Research, Maryland, USA
(https://ccr.cancer.gov/Surgery-Branch/steven-a-rosenberg)

[111] 'Remarkable' therapy beats terminal breast cancer, *4th June 2018 (James Gallagher, Health Correspondent, BBC News)*

the most highly personalised treatment imaginable. It remains experimental and still requires considerably more testing before it can be used more widely.

It starts by analysing the DNA of a tumour to identify what might make the cancer cells visible to the immune system. Then the patient's white blood cells are screened and those capable of attacking the cancer are extracted and grown in huge quantities in the laboratory.

Dr. Rosenberg did just that before he injected 90 billion of these cells into a 49-year old patient who had terminal Stage IV breast cancer that had metastasised to tennis ball size tumours in her liver and more all over her body. The cancer disappeared totally within 30 days.

It is a truly remarkable achievement in itself but it is even more remarkable that five years later there is no sign of cancer in the patient's body. Yet, Dr. Rosenberg warns, "This is highly experimental and we're just learning how to do this, but potentially it is applicable to any cancer. A lot of work needs to be done, but the potential exists for a paradigm shift in cancer therapy - a unique drug for every cancer patient - it is very different to any other kind of treatment."

The Australian Haematologist / Oncologist Glenn Begley agreed with Dr. Rosenberg when he raised the question of why we haven't cured cancer yet in his lecture 'The Complex Biology of Cancer' [112]. He stated that a successful cure depends on the recognition of the inner workings of cancer cells because cancer is not just one disease but that every cancer is different.

Dr. Begley stated that the growth of a tumour reflects years of on-going evolutionary selection and is only detected very late in its development. Cancer starts in a single cell and

---

[112] Prof. Dr. Glenn Begley, Haematologist / Oncologist, University of Melbourne, Australia
(The Complex Biology of Cancer - TEDx)

although multiple changes in genes occur during its growth, tumours still share 99.9% of their genetic identity with healthy cells. It implies that tumour evolution is ongoing and that the main tumour does not kill the cancer patient but the metastases.

In short, when the migration and spread of cancer cells to other organs is not stopped in time, it will kill the patient. He is in agreement with Leonard Sender that billions of cancer cells are floating around in our bodies. In his opinion the remission of cancer is achieved when the count of cancer cells is lowered to less than 1 billion. A relapse or recurrence of cancer occurs when the number of cancer cells rises above 1 billion. That is the reason why adjunct and adjuvant therapies should aim for the treatment of micro-metastases because the time for therapeutic intervention is very limited.

Despite progress in basic research that has resulted in a better understanding of tumour biology and led to the design of new generations of targeted cancer drugs, recent large clinical trials of new chemotherapeutic drugs have not resulted in relevant differences in treatment outcomes.

Moreover, the number of approved chemotherapy drugs with any level of proven efficacy is disappointingly low. Dr. Aida Karachi writes that the failure of the conventional cancer therapeutics of surgical resection, radio- and chemotherapy has led to an increasing interest in immunotherapy that is enhancing immune system responses to fight cancer cells.

She states that monoclonal antibodies, immune checkpoint blockades, targeted therapy, and adoptive cell therapy are currently part of the immunotherapy armamentarium and claims that immunotherapy has "tremendous" success in the treatment of cancers and is considered as a standard care of treatment and recurrence preventive therapy for a variety of cancers.

The White Blood Cell Phenomenon

Aida Karachi states in her report *Immunotherapy for Treatment of Cancer* that "the failure of currently available therapeutics for cancers, has led to increasing interest in immunotherapy for cancer treatment. [It] harnesses the patients' immune system to kill cancer cells thereby avoiding toxic effects of traditional chemotherapy and radiotherapy."

It has been known for a long time that the immune system is capable of attacking cancer cells. Its white blood cells play the crucial part in immunotherapy. It sets in motion a complex defence mechanism based primarily on lymphocytes, i.e. the white blood cells T-cells, B-cells, and NK-cells. They recognise when a body cell is infected by a pathogen and destroy it. T-cells also activate B-cells to produce antibodies.

Antibodies are proteins called immunoglobulins present in the serum and cells of the immune system. There are five different types of it named IgM, IgA, IgG, IgE, and IgD. Each of these plays a different role in the immune system. Using the lock and key principle, antibodies usually fit certain pathogens. They have different capabilities and occur at different stages in response to encountering a pathogen.

IgM antibodies are found mainly in the blood and lymph fluid and are the first to appear in response to the initial exposure to a pathogen.

IgA antibodies attach to pathogens more strongly and are mainly found in the mucous membranes of the respiratory tract and the digestive system.

IgG antibodies are the most common antibody found in the bloodstream and other body fluids with approximately 80% of immunoglobulins. They protect mainly against bacterial and viral infections.

IgE antibodies are normally found only in small amounts in the bloodstream but increase in reaction to allergies or an infection from parasites.

IgD antibodies are mostly found on the surface of B-cells and help to regulate its function. The function of IgD antibodies circulating in the blood is unknown.

The three types of white blood cells, T-cells, B-cells, and NK-cells have distinctly different functions. The following are brief introductions to their origins, functions, and fate.

T-cells[113]

A T-cell plays the central role in the immune response. It originates from the haematopoietic[114] stem cells in the bone marrow. It is a type of lymphocyte, which migrates from the bone marrow to the thymus gland where it matures.

After its release from the thymus gland it goes from naïve to memory cell in a whole continuum of development in the peripheral tissue, circulating in the blood, or the lymphatic system.

Once stimulated by an antigen, a T-cell secretes chemical messenger molecules called cytokines, which stimulate the differentiation of B-cells into antibody producing cells.

The more often a T-cell becomes activated by an antigen or pathogen signal, the further along the line of memory development it is and the faster it responds to that specific signal.

Groups of specific, differentiated T-cells have an important role in controlling and shaping the immune response by providing a variety of immune-related functions.

One of these functions is immune-mediated cancer cell death that is carried out by T-cells.

---

[113] Immunotherapy for Treatment of Cancer
Aida Karachi, 11th May 2018
(https://www.intechopen.com/books/current-trends-in-cancer-management/immunotherapy-for-treatment-of-cancer)

[114] haematopoietic, adj. of haemopoiesis - the production of blood cells and platelets, which occurs in the bone marrow.

A typical T-cell may have as many as 20,000 receptor molecules on its membrane surface. They consist of two polypeptide chains[115]. Many are unique receptors that enable the T-cell to respond to virtually any antigen or pathogen. A cytotoxic T-cell, activated by various cytokines, binds to and kills infected cells and cancer cells.

Adoptive T-cell therapy (ACT) is a treatment to enhance the T-cells' ability to kill cancer cells by infusing a patient with a multiple of immune system derived cells that originate from the patient. Both peripheral blood T-cells and tumour infiltrating lymphocytes extracted from tumours are utilised to generate specific T-cells for ACT. These cancer-reactive T-cells are multiplied by the billions in a laboratory and then directly infused back into the patient.

In cancer treatment, T-cells are constantly exposed to antigen stimulation, which results in a gradual deterioration of their function with a persistent increase of inhibitory receptors and by losing the cytokine production ability. These defects are defined as exhaustion. Inhibitory receptors are encountered in high quantities on exhausted T-cells, while the high number of inhibitory ligands on cancer cells increases the chance of T-cell exhaustion.

B-cells[116]

B-cells represent about 5–15% of circulating blood lymphocytes and are responsible for the humoral immune response, as a critical component of the adaptive immune system. Their roles are not limited only to the production of antigen-specific antibodies but also to antigen presentation.

---

[115] polypeptide chains - a linear organic polymer consisting of a large number of amino-acid residues bonded together in a chain, forming part of a protein molecule.

[116] Introductory Chapter: B-Cells
Mourad Aribi, 26th Feb. 2020
(https://www.intechopen.com/books/normal-and-malignant-b-cell/introductory-chapter-b-cells)

This allows them to interact with cells involved in cell-mediated immunity and produce cytokines within immunological synapses (IS).

Antibodies allow B-cells to provide systemic protection of the host and immune surveillance through pathogen recognition and organisation of immune reactions. Their expression varies according to the state of differentiation of B-cells.

After activation, B-cells transform into plasma cells that secrete antibodies of the same specificity as their membrane B-cell antigen receptor complex. Secreted antibodies are transported rapidly throughout the body by blood or lymph or secreted through the epithelia, the thin tissue of the outer layer of a surface or lining of hollow structures, to protect the interface between the body and its environment.

Knowing that all cells develop from the early lymphoid progenitors that originate from totipotent[117] haematopoietic stem cells, cell fate results from several lineage choices. The B-cell progenitors continue to develop in the bone marrow.

B-cells are threatened by various pathologies, including
(i)   immune system deficiency
(ii) autoimmune disorders, and
(iii) allergies that are particularly related to regulatory abnormalities.

NK-cells[118]

An NK-cell is a lymphocyte that originates in the bone marrow and develops without the influence of the thymus. It attaches to a tumour or cancer cell, releases chemicals that breach the cell wall, and causes its apoptosis. But more than

---

[117] totipotent - an immature cell capable of giving rise to any cell type.
[118] NK Cells and Cancer
May Sabry and Mark W. Lowdell, 13th Dec. 2017
(https://www.intechopen.com/books/natural-killer-cells/nk-cells-and-cancer)

that, it exerts cytotoxicity and secretes a wide variety of cytokines to inhibit tumour progression.

NK-cells play a critical role in tumour control and eradication. A long-term epidemiological study following cancer patients reported that subjects with low NK-cell activity had a high incidence of several types of cancer. The NK-cells' two main effector functions against tumour targets are target cell elimination and cytokine secretion.

The contents of the NK-cell granules released for target cell elimination contain the critical effector molecules perforin, which is a membrane disrupting protein, and serine proteases. Perforin results in the disruption of internal trafficking and binds to phospholipid components of the lipid bilayer to facilitate entry of the serine proteases into the target cell that induce the target cell's apoptosis.

Even resting NK-cells secrete a plethora of cytokines that help eliminate target cells and amplify activation signals for a more efficient immune response. NK-cell stimulation results in enhanced secretion of cytokines, which in turn influence the activity of the other immune cells.

NK-cells require the co-engagement of multiple activating receptors in order to exhibit natural cytotoxicity against tumour target cells. Upon an encounter with potential target cells, an immunological synapse forms at the point of contact between the NK-cell and the target cell, where NK-cell receptors can interact with their respective ligands. Given sufficient activation signals, NK-cell cytoskeletal rearrangements are initiated, which result in the polarisation of NK-cell lytic granules toward the immunological synapse, where they eventually fuse and release their cytotoxic contents onto the target cell.

The ability of NK-cells to kill tumour cells has made them attractive in immunotherapy. NK-cell impairments associated with tumour development and progression have been frequently reported in cancer patients, including weakened effector functions and an altered phenotype with down-regulation of activating NK-cell receptors. Different strategies have been employed to repair, replace, or enhance the biological functions of autologous or allogeneic NK-cells *in vivo* and *ex vivo*. In a clinical setting, the key factors to be considered are the number, purity, proliferative capacity, and activation state of NK-cells. The most limiting of these factors is obtaining a sufficient number of NK-cells, hence the extensive development of *ex vivo* expansion for NK-cell adoptive immunotherapy applications.

The last three decades unravelled different molecular mechanisms governing NK-cell-mediated anti-tumour functions. This led to the development of a variety of strategies for NK-cell-based immunotherapy of cancer. However, many challenges still remain as the molecular and functional characterisation of NK-cells and their receptors is improved, and the different signalling pathways involved in NK-cell recognition of targets are deciphered.

Conclusion:
It is crucial to be aware of the white blood cells' function in the immune system to understand why a healthy and strong immune system is so important not just to defeat cancer but any pathogen including viruses and toxic microorganisms.

Immunotherapies in Use Today

The following are some of immunotherapies that are used today on a limited or experimental basis:

- Non-Specific Immune Stimulation Therapy is the original immunotherapy that Dr. Coley used by chance in 1891. It doesn't target cancer cells specifically but boosts the patient's immune system in a more general way by using a family of molecules known as cytokines. These molecules, produced by the cells of the immune system, control the activity of other immunity cells and lead to a better immune response. Interferon and interleukin, two types of cytokine, are able to stimulate the growth of white blood cells and thus boost the complete immune system. The activation increases the probability of the immune system to attack cancer cells and rid the patient's body of cancer.[119]

Side effects:
Nausea and fever.

- T-cell Transfer Therapy is a type of immunotherapy still in its experimental stage that boosts specific parts of the immune system and thus enables the immune cells to attack cancer cells. T-cells are collected, grown millionfold in a lab, and injected back into the bloodstream of the patient.[120]

There are two types of T-cell transfer therapy:
- The tumour-infiltrating lymphocytes therapy (TIL) involves immune system T-cells found inside a cancer tumour. They are not numerous enough to overcome the tumour's ability to block the immune system. Extracted from the cancer tumour they are multiplied millionfold in a laboratory and subjecting them to Interleukin-2,

---

[119] Non-specific immune stimulation
(*institut-curie.org/dossier-pedagogique/non-specific-immunotherapy-stimulating-immune-system*)

[120] T-cell Transfer Therapy
(*https://www.cancer.gov/aboutcancer/treatment/types/immunotherapy/t-cell-transfer-therapy*)

which is a signalling molecule of the immune system that regulates the activities of white blood cells responsible for immunity. Injected into the bloodstream, these lymphocytes can overcome the blockage of the immune system and eradicate the tumours.

Side effects:
TIL may cause capillary leak syndrome, which releases fluids and proteins from blood vessels into surrounding tissue and may lead to multiple organ failure and death.

- The CAR T-cell therapy uses extracted white blood cells that are genetically modified to contain a protein known as chimeric antigen receptor (CAR) and then multiplied in the lab. This CAR protein allows the T-cell to attach itself to receptors of a cancer tumour, which improves its ability to kill the tumour. This therapy is only approved for blood cancer treatment.

Side effects:
The CAR T-cells released into the bloodstream release a large number of cytokines. Their sudden increase may cause fever, nausea, headache, rapid heartbeat, low blood pressure, and trouble breathing with the potential of death due to a catastrophic autoimmune response.

Note: The FDA (US Food and Drug Administration) put a clinical hold on CAR T-cell programs in 2018 until further notice and suspended new clinical trials because of safety concerns.

• Immune Checkpoint Inhibitor Therapy [121] helps immune checkpoints on cell surfaces to control an immune response. The checkpoint protein PD-1 keeps a T-cell from attacking a healthy cell when it binds with the healthy cell's PD-L1 checkpoint protein that tells the T-cell to leave it

---

[121] Immune Checkpoint Inhibitors
(https://www.mdanderson.org/treatment-options/immune-checkpoint-inhibitors.html)

alone. But cancer cells use these PD-L1 checkpoints as well to avoid being detected.

Immune Checkpoint Inhibitors are drugs that block these checkpoints and allow the T-cells to kill the cancer cell. There are a number of PD-1 as well as PD-L1 inhibitor drugs on the market that block the binding and help the immune system response to kill cancer cells. No explanation can be found if these drugs differentiate at all between the checkpoint inhibitors of healthy and cancer cells or if it is just a case of the healthy cells being so much more numerous than cancer cells, even in patients with advanced Stage IV cancer, that the apoptosis of healthy cells is simply considered a matter of collateral damage with a good chance of survival for the patient.

Side effects:
These drugs allow the immune system to attack healthy cells that can cause various organs like the lung, liver, and kidneys to malfunction that are otherwise unaffected by cancer and result in the death of the patient. This therapy only works in 10 - 15% of patients treated.

- Personalised Cancer Treatment Vaccines are the latest targets in the quest for finding the panacea that will provide a cure for cancer. While the research of cancer prevention vaccines that strengthen the body's natural defences against the development of cancer is very much at an experimental stage, the cancer vaccines that attack cancer tumours and have been developed so far show some promise to be effective. In particular a vaccine made from a patient's own antigen presenting autologous dendritic cells (a type of white blood cell) has been approved by the FDA for the treatment of advanced prostate cancer. It is used to kill existing cancer cells but has not yet been shown to provide a cure and prevent the recurrence of cancer.

A vaccine for all types of cancer is still a long way off but the recent developments show that the scientists involved in the cancer research and vaccine development are on the right track.[122]

- Anti-angiogenic therapy[123] is an approach of achieving the apoptosis of cancer cells by preventing the development of new blood vessels. The growth and metastasis of a tumour depends upon the steady supply of nutrients, which are delivered via the vascular system.

Solid malignant tumours develop a network of blood vessels that assures its growth with the steady supply of nutrients. Anti-angiogenic therapies prevent and reverse this network. The results of the present studies suggest that the combination of angiogenesis inhibitors and cytotoxic chemotherapy agents may produce a synergistic therapeutic effect in the apoptosis of cancer cells.

Side effects:
All the presently approved angiogenesis inhibitor medications produce severe side effects ranging from the swelling of face and tongue, skin blistering and peeling, lung, liver and kidney malfunction to gastrointestinal perforation that can result in the death of the patient. The exception is a medication developed in China that is still undergoing Phase III clinical trials. Cancer is caused in one third of all cases by diet. As an alternative to medical treatment, it is recommended to switch to anti-angiogenic foods rich in vitamin E such as olive oil, green leafy vegetables, walnuts, and pine nuts as well as Earl Grey tea, glucosamine, citrus fruits, red grapes, berries, garlic, and parsley and cut back on carbohydrates.

---

[122] Personalized Cancer Vaccines in Clinical Trials
(The Scientist, Jasreet Hundal and Elaine R. Mardis, Jul 15, 2019)

[123] Anti-angiogenic therapy for cancer: An update
(Belal Al-Husein, Maha Abdalla, Morgan Trepte, Davaid L. DeRemer, and Payaningal R. Somanath, National Center for Biotechnology Information, U.S. National Library of Medicine)

Summary: The side effects of the immunotherapies with the exception of Non-Specific Immune Stimulation Therapy provide proof of the early stage of the ongoing research despite some positive results. Once the side effects can be avoided or overcome, then the goal of eradicating cancer without harming healthy cells, tissue, and organs could be within reach.

What's New, Doc?

A vast number of researchers, scientists, oncologists, and patients look to immunotherapy as the most promising development in the struggle of finding a cure for cancer. Several researchers have gone public with results that are very encouraging. It has to be stated, though, that many of the results are not final or proven over a lengthy period in extended empirical clinical trials. But what the researchers found out was nevertheless encouraging.

Prof. Carlo Maley[124] stated that slowing down the growth of cancer would be a major step forward to bring down the mortality of people stricken with cancer. In his research the first mutations that start the cancerous process happen up to 50 years before cancer is detected. If this process could be slowed down by a factor of two, cancer would only occur way beyond a person's normal life expectancy. He investigated the use of the anti-inflammatory drug Aspirin and his research showed that it slowed the mutations by a factor of ten in the people that took this drug. He noted as well the strengthening of the tumour suppressor cells P53 lead to the apoptosis of cancer and damaged cells.

In his pursuit of cancer research, Dr. Michael Jensen[125] was shocked that cancer clinics still rely on the antiquated therapies of surgery, chemo- and radiotherapy. These therapies are not smart enough to eliminate cancer cells and leave healthy body parts unharmed. His research includes molecular biology, genetic engineering, and protein use. He states, the cure for cancer is already in our bodies - our immune system. His research focuses on cytotoxic T-cells, the white blood cells responsible for eliminating cancer.

---

[124] How Nature has already beaten Cancer
Prof. Carlo Maley, Cancer Biologist, Arizona State University

[125] Immune to Cancer, *Dr. Michael Jensen, Director of the Ben Towne Center for Childhood Cancer Research, Seattle Children's Research Institute*

He overcame the problem of cancer cells making themselves invisible by "re-programming cancer specific T-cells". He isolated immune cells from a blood sample, reprogrammed them with a DNA molecule to enable them to detect proteins only present in cancer cells, then multiplied these cells to a few billion, and injected them into the patient where they eradicate cancer cells and leave healthy cells intact. The reprogrammed cells will stay in the body for the life of the patient and continue eradicating any cancer cell. Dr. Jensen claims a 91% success rate with his treatment, a form of adoptive cell therapy. However, to date his therapy is limited to treating leukaemia.

Prof. Matt Trau,[126] a chemist and bioengineer involved in the development of nano-diagnostics, was a member of a team treating a patient with the unorthodox method of administering a non-specific skin cancer medication for the patient's melanoma. The therapy yielded the result of the patient being in complete remission but the young woman died four weeks later from heart failure. Her preceding aggressive treatment with chemotherapy had weakened her heart so badly that it stopped functioning.

Prof. Trau states that this outcome could have been prevented had the patient been monitored with nano-diagnostics, a technology used to refine the discovery of biomarkers during her chemotherapy and the treatment stopped when no progress or a worsening of her condition had been registered.

The malfunction of organs not related to cancer due to the effects of chemo- and radiotherapy has been noted and documented by many other medical scientists and practitioners all over the world.

---

[126] An End to Cancer Mortality with Nano-Diagnostics, *Prof. Matt Trau, Professor of Chemistry, The University of Queensland, Deputy Director of the Australian Institute for Bioengineering and Nanotechnology*

CRISPR - Not a New Potato Chip

Contrary to the first impression one might have upon hearing CRISPR mentioned, it is not something you find in the grocery store among the assortment of potato crisps, as Minesh Khatri, MD,[127] points out. It is a technology that gives scientists the ability to change an organism's DNA. It is the simplest, fastest, and most accurate technique of gene editing.

That shouldn't come as a surprise since it was so to speak 'invented' by Mother Nature as a genome editing system in bacteria from where it was adapted. It works as follows: the bacteria catch a snippet of DNA of an invading pathogen and create an array that allows to recognise it, cut its DNA and thus disable or destroy it. Simplicity in action!

CRISPR is the acronym for "clustered regularly interspaced short palindromic repeat". A Cas9 protein (CRISPR-associated protein 9)[128] is added to a cell with a piece of RNA that is present in living cells. It then moves along the DNA of the pathogen until it finds and binds to a 20-DNA-letter sequence that matches the RNA sequence out of the six billion letters in each cell, cuts the DNA at the target, and introduces mutations that disable the gene.

Once this action had been recognised, it was widely used to edit the genomes of plants and animals. Lately, the research has focused on the potential treatment of a variety of diseases in humans but it has to be determined still whether genome editing is safe and effective for use in humans.

One important area of exploration is immunotherapy to enable the body's immune system to eradicate cancer cells and tumours.

---

[127] What Is CRISPR?
Minesh Khatri, MD, assistant professor of medicine, Columbia University, 14th Oct. 2019
(https://www.webmd.com/cancer/crispr-facts-overview#1)

[128] The Cas9 protein derived from type II CRISPR bacterial immune systems serves to cut DNA to alter a cell's genome.

The technology developed so far lets scientists cut and paste bits of DNA of genes to alter their traits with the aim of curing diseases. Its 'aim' to cure diseases is a clear indication that this technology is still in its infancy.

The big problem in regard to cancer immunotherapy is the safe alteration of T-cells to chase down and eradicate cancer cells and tumours without causing them to destroy healthy cells. All types of cancer are linked to problems in genes and CRISPR holds the promise of fixing these problems, though there are no treatments or cures yet.

It works by identifying a specific strand of the DNA of a T-cell, replacing it by "cutting" the original DNA and "pasting" in replacement DNA that enables it to recognise and eradicate cancer cells. It sounds simple enough but there are many inherent risks that raise many questions. Khatri states that there is a chance for example of accidentally editing a very similar DNA that is not the target. Even a minor change in DNA can have big impacts and researchers need to use a lot of caution. Also, they don't know yet what side effects it may have. There are several Phase I trials targeting cancer and so far they showed CRISPR to be safe. That is encouraging but it is a long way to go from these trials to safe, effective treatments.

Another aspect of altering genes concerns the research of not just treating and eradicating cancer but also preventing the disease from happening. That is an enormously large area of research because it involves the investigation of historical cancer data, the biopsies of cancer tumours of the parents and grandparents of a child, and then finding in the child a genetic flaw that might indicate the occurrence of cancer at a later age. It is a very ambitious undertaking and there won't be a simple solution. Nevertheless, it is highly commendable that scientists are targeting the prevention of cancer at this still early stage of the development of CRISPR for cancer immunotherapy.

Cold Plasma Cancer Immunotherapy

In stark contrast to individuals promoting unorthodox immunotherapies stands the research of Cold Atmospheric Plasma (CAP) cancer immunotherapy. In a spirit of global collaboration was the 6th International Workshop on Plasma for Cancer Treatment 2019 held in Antwerp, [129] Belgium. Researchers from France, Japan, Spain, Germany, South Korea, USA, and the host country discussed the latest developments of cold plasma cancer therapy.

They contributed with their research results of plasma sources and plasma equipment used for cancer treatment, plasma-cancer interactions, destruction of cancer cells by plasma, mechanisms of plasma selectivity towards cancer cells, plasma-liquid interaction, plasma chemistry in biological liquids, and clinical and animal studies of cancer treatment by plasma. Despite the advances of the technology and the encouraging results of this revolutionary therapy, the participants concluded that CAP cancer immunotherapy is still at a stage of early development.

Prof. Annemie Bogaerts [130] heads a research group that investigates plasma medicine while focussing on cold plasma for cancer treatment that offers the possibility to selectively eliminate cancer cells while leaving surrounding, normal cells, unaffected. But she stated like many of her colleagues that the mechanisms underlying the CAP selectivity towards cancer cells are not yet fully understood.

"Plasma creates a cocktail of reactive species, such as electrons, ions and radicals, besides neutral gas molecules, which makes it useful for various applications," said Bogaerts. "The reactive oxygen and nitrogen species produced are

---

[129] 6th International Workshop on Plasma for Cancer Treatment - 2019 (https://www.uantwerpen.be/en/conferences/plasma-for-cancer-treatment-iwpct/)

[130] Prof. Annemie Bogaerts, Dept. of Chemistry, University of Antwerp, Belgium

190

thought to be responsible for the biological effects to cells and are important for cancer treatment."

What is plasma? Plasma is an ionised gas such as helium, argon, heliox,[131] or air that carries an electric charge after losing some of its electrons by heat or via an electromagnetic field. It has been defined as one of the four states of matter: solid, liquid, gas, and plasma.

In thermal hot plasmas the majority of the electron particles are ionised and temperatures reach extremely high levels. Hot plasma is found in its uncontrolled form on the surface of the sun or in a controlled form in a plasma-torch that is used in manufacturing industries for high-precision metal cutting.

In cold plasma, on the other hand, only a few of the particles are ionised with a relatively high voltage difference between two points. As a result, it maintains a temperature of about 25 to 37° Celsius between room temperature and body temperature, which makes it suitable for use in medical applications. When the voltage is applied, the neutral particles of the gas are ionised by removing one or more electrons in the electric field and the result is cold plasma. Needed for this process is a bottle of pressurised gas, wires, an electrode, an anode, electricity, a retainer space for the plasma, and a device to apply the cold plasma.

How did it all start? One has to go back all the way to 1857 when Ernst Werner von Siemens[132] first reported an ozone production discharge. He had constructed a dielectric-barrier discharge contraption with one of two steel electrode plates covered with the dielectric barrier material mica, a silicate mineral used as a thermal or electrical insulator. He charged the device with high voltage alternating current, used argon as

---

[131] Heliox is a gas mixture of 80% helium and 20% oxygen that is used in the treatment of patients with breathing problems

[132] Ernst Werner von Siemens, electrical engineer, inventor, and industrialist. 13th Dec. 1816 - 6th Dec. 1892

the working gas, and saw the bright blue filaments between the two plates.

The investigation of the ozone discharge that is now called cold plasma was continued some twenty years later by Sir William Crookes[133] who identified it as the fourth state of matter in 1879. That was the beginning of plasma research but it took many years until cold plasma's usefulness in medicine generally and cancer therapy specifically was discovered and began to be used. It was not until the 1990s that cold plasma became the subject of intensified research for medical applications. Its capacity to kill bacteria was well known but the large dielectric-barrier discharge (DBD) system used to disinfect materials, instruments, and critical areas in hospitals turned out to be impractical for biomedical applications.

In 1998 Prof. Mounir Laroussi[134] had the idea of a device that emits a single low temperature atmospheric pressure plume of cold plasma that could be used in the medical treatment of wounds and the disinfection of the oral cavity in dentistry. Together with his assistant Xin Pei Lu, a postdoctoral researcher at the Frank Reidy Research Center of the Old Dominion University in Norfolk, Virginia, he developed a 12.5cm (5") long and 1.5cm (1") diameter handheld device that produces a single plume of cold plasma up to 3cm (2") in length. That was a major breakthrough and received the laudation it deserved in 2005.

Since then the development of instruments used for different applications has picked up the pace and already some of them have gone through lengthy clinical trials.

How does CAP actually work? In medical applications there are two approaches, the indirect and the direct discharge of the plasma. The indirect discharge with a dielectric barrier

---

[133] Sir William Crookes, British chemist and physicist
17th June 1832 - 4th April 1919

[134] Prof. Mounir Laroussi, electrical and computer engineering
Old Dominion University, Norfolk, Virginia, USA

discharge allows the plasma to flow from the main discharge arc from the anode to the cathode where the target area is located between the two electrodes. In the application of the direct discharge, the device that emits the cold plasma contains the anode as well as the cathode, while the area of treatment, the living tissue of a wound or cancer cell, for example, is one of the electrodes. [135]

Cold plasma is anti-microbial and its application has the immediate effect of killing practically 100% of bacteria, viruses, and fungi, while at the same time stimulating the growth of healthy cells and the immune system cells. It increases the blood supply to the vessels and thus the reactive oxygen to a level that is lethal to tumours and cancer cells.

The plasma pencil is still mainly used in treating chronic wounds but more areas of application are subject to trials including cancer immunotherapy. In all treatments conducted so far there have been no side effects detected.

At Greifswald University [136] in northern Germany it was discovered by coincidence in 2007 that cold plasma also caused the apoptosis of cancer cells when a superficial wound was treated with cold atmospheric plasma and the subcutaneous cancer cells underneath the wound were eradicated. The experimental treatment of skin cancer worked very well. From there it was a natural progression to explore

---

[135] Molecular Mechanisms of the Efficacy of Cold Atmospheric Pressure Plasma (CAP) in Cancer Treatment
Marie Luise Semmler, Sander Bekeschus, Mirijam Schäfer, Thoralf Bernhardt, Tobias Fischer, Katharina Witzke, Christian Seebauer, Henrike Rebl, Eberhard Grambow, Brigitte Vollmar, J. Barbara Nebe, Hans-Robert Metelmann, Thomas von Woedtke, Steffen Emmert and Lars Boeckmann
(https://www.researchgate.net/publication/338814878_Molecular_Me chanisms_of_the_Efficacy_of_Cold_Atmospheric_Pressure_Plasma_ CAP_in_Cancer_Treatment)

[136] Universität Greifswald, public research university in Greifswald, Mecklenburg-Vorpommern, Germany
(https://physik.uni-greifswald.de/en/research/)

the effect of CAP on other types of the disease such as brain, breast, lung, and cervical cancer.

As a consequence of the successful eradication of skin cancer new devices are being considered for development at the Greifswald University such as an instrument similar to an endoscope that can be used for CAP treatment of cancer of internal organs.

In his pursuit of making the application of cold plasma simpler, Dr. Carsten Mahrenholz[137] developed together with the Leibniz Institute for Plasma Research a plasma cube and silicon plasma patch to treat chronic wounds that accelerate the healing process and improve the immune system.

The cube generates plasma that is emitted into the patch, which is applied like a sticky plaster to the treatment area and can replace the use of antibiotics. If the plasma patch will also cause the apoptosis or necrosis of subcutaneous cancer cells is still under investigation.

"Although studies have shown that cancer cells die quicker than normal cells with cold plasma, this is still in very early stages so we have to be humble about whether cold plasma can actually treat cancer," says Mahrenholz.[138]

"Nevertheless, scientifically, this is an interesting field and I hope we can someday help cancer patients beyond the benefit of palliation with this promising new technology."

---

[137] Dr. Carsten Mahrenholz, co-founder and CEO of coldplasmatech (https://eithealth.eu/project/coldplasmatech/)

[138] Activating a liquid with plasma gives it anti-cancer properties, *Julianna Photopoulos, Horizon: The EU Research & Innovation Magazine, 26th July 2018 (https://medicalxpress.com/news/2018-07-liquid-plasma-anti-cancer-properties.html)*

Immunotherapy: An Old Hat?

While immense research is going on around the world to find a reliable therapy that will strengthen the immune system and eradicate cancer cells without toxic chemicals, it is not a new concept at all. The first time it was applied very successfully was by the orthopaedic surgeon and cancer researcher William B. Coley in New York in 1891.

He had observed cancerous growths that disappeared after patients had been infected with streptococcus bacteria. Reviewing research papers, he learned that Sir James Paget[139] in Britain in 1853 and Prof. Karl Wilhelm Busch [140] in Germany in 1866 had observed similar developments and were certain that bacterial infections stimulated the immune system, which caused the regression and disappearance of tumours. When a man came to Dr. Coley with a growth on his throat that hindered him eating and even breathing properly, he infected him with live streptococcus bacteria. Within days the growth, a cancer tumour started to shrink and disappeared soon thereafter.

What Dr. Coley had done, without being fully aware of the consequences, was to put the patient's immune system with the bacteria into 'overdrive', so to speak, that was then strong enough to tackle the tumour.

Immunologists today know that the injection of streptococcus bacteria immediately caused a massive increase of white blood cells that strengthened the immune system to the point of being capable of attacking the cancerous growth and causing its apoptosis. Yet when Coley published his

---

[139] Sir James Paget, English surgeon and pathologist, with Rudolf Virchow one of the founders of scientific medical pathology
(https://en.wikipedia.org/wiki/James_Paget)

[140] Karl David Wilhelm Busch, Surgeon, Surgical Clinic of the University of Bonn, the world's first institution investigating cancer immunotherapy.
(https://en.wikipedia.org/wiki/Wilhelm_Busch_(surgeon))

therapy, nobody took him seriously - not at least because little was known about the origin and function of cancer at that time.

This first example of immunotherapy would have been all but forgotten had it not been for his daughter Dr. Helen Coley who doggedly persisted that there was more to her father's cancer treatment then was generally believed.

She founded the non-profit Cancer Research Institute together with Oliver R. Grace in 1954. Her research together with her collaborator Dr. Lloyd J. Old yielded the discovery of checkpoints on blood cells and immunotherapy was on its way to be taken seriously.

The Cancer Research Institute (CRI) is not as its name implies a research institute but a funding body for the research conducted by other institutes and organisations that focus on immunological cancer treatments, rather than conventional surgery and chemo- and radiotherapy.

The CRI spends about 75% of its funding on research and clinical trials for immunotherapies and 12% on education and scientific conferences.

Cancer Vaccine - Not A Dream Any Longer

CRI announced its partnership with the biopharmaceutical company CureVac located in Tübingen, Germany, in 2013 to enable clinical testing of a messenger ribonucleic acid (mRNA) novel cancer immunotherapy vaccine treatment option.[141] Ludwig Cancer Research and Boehringer Ingelheim have since entered this arrangement in support of the research of vaccines for five types of cancer - advanced melanoma, adenoid cystic carcinoma, and cancers of the head and neck - that have passed the discovery and development phases and are undergoing Phase I clinical trials.

CureVac's cancer research is based on its proprietary mRNA platform that enhances antigenic properties of proteins and triggers the patient's immune system to attack cancer cells. It simulates a viral infection that stimulates the immune system to recognise cancer cells, leading to immune-mediated killing of both infected and non-infected cancer cells.

The mRNA cancer vaccines guide the immune system to target tumour neo-antigens for an anti-cancer immune response. It involves the design of mRNA molecules capable of orchestrating immune attacks against neo-antigens and thus recognising and eradicating cancer cells. The cancer vaccine immunology strategy is to direct the immune system to recognise cancers, which don't respond to current immunotherapy treatments.

One of the company's partners stated, "Firing up the patient's immune system to attack the tumours is the most precise approach to cancer treatment. The research done today, will deliver breakthrough treatments in the future."

It is noteworthy that mRNA has been known for several decades but its therapeutic potential was not recognised until

---

[141] CureVac Collaborates with CRI and Ludwig to Enable Immunotherapy Clinical Testing, *4th Nov. 2013* *(https://www.cancerresearch.org/news/2013/curevac-collaborates-cri-ludwig-clinical-testing)*

the biomedical researcher Ingmar Hoerr discovered in the late 1990s that it could be injected directly into tissue as a vaccine to fire up the immune system. Hoerr founded CureVac, the company that was the first to use mRNA for a successful therapeutic purpose.

Firing up the immune system has been recognised as the effective method to combat cancer. Various approaches have been taken in the recent past including conventional protective vaccination of weakened pathogens reproducing to a limited extent. The immune system reacts to these pathogens, forms protective antibodies, and stores the immune response in the T-cell "memory", which allows the immune system to react faster and more effectively when it comes into contact with the pathogen again. Also, protein-based vaccines of the pathogen are introduced as an antigen, against which the immune system forms an immune response. In vector vaccines, a harmless virus is used to introduce and produce mRNA as an antigen in body cells. These vaccines proved to be effective in strengthening the immune system and contribute to the early detection of cancer cells but not the eradication of cancer tumours.

Therefore, the research focus shifted to RNA and DNA vaccines that contain genetic information of cancer tumours. They aim to trigger a defence reaction of the immune system to eradicate cancer tumours.

RNA vaccines are made up of mRNA that contains instructions for T-cells and B-cells to form antigens, i.e. virus proteins to provoke an immune response. mRNA vaccines are not transported into the cell nucleus. Therefore, there is no risk that it will be integrated into the genome of body cells.

DNA vaccines work similarly. However, the DNA molecule is introduced into the cell nucleus and read there in the form of mRNA, which migrates out of the cell nucleus and is then translated into antigen. It has been feared that the DNA brought into the cell is introduced into the actual genetic material of the host cell and can cause increased tumour formation or autoimmune diseases. Yet, no such development has ever been proven or observed.

Since the research and development of five different mRNA vaccines have been going strong for the past years, I am quite hopeful that a cancer immunotherapy vaccine final trial will be announced in the not too distant future. But a lot of work over several years lies ahead until such final phase clinical trial of these potent mRNA cancer vaccines will be conducted and completed. But once it is done, it will be equivalent to a quantum leap in cancer immunotherapy.

Several more biopharmaceutical companies have jumped on what can be considered by now the mRNA bandwagon in the USA, Germany, Switzerland, China, India, and more.

The unsettling aspect of this otherwise very welcome development of competition to see who comes first in the eradication of cancer tumours is the fact that most of these innovative and pioneering biopharmaceutical companies have already tied themselves for comparatively paltry investments to Big Pharma.

That raises questions about the outcome of the vaccine development: Will the Big Pharma investors insist that the vaccine cannot be a permanent cure but only a temporary fix to assure them of massive profits for eternity? What price will they insist on charging for an effective vaccine once full-scale industrial production has been ramped up? Will their greed be satisfied with less than a million bucks per shot?

One has to anticipate that my dream scenario of $200 for a treatment to cure you of cancer for good will remain but a dream scenario and the scourge of cancer will stay with humanity forever - if Big Pharma can help it.

The Outlook for Immunotherapy

Conventional cancer therapy, even the most ardent defenders of cut, burn, and poison admit, does not provide a cure for cancer. It only palliates and provides at best a life extension of a few days, months, or years. It is also a vastly complex procedure that is very expensive and most often extremely painful for the patients.

Despite the proclaimed advances of the treatment of a very limited number of cancers, most of the more than 200 types of cancer cannot be treated with the conventional therapy at all or with any degree of success or hope for a limited time of progression free survival. Due to the nature of cancer, the conventional treatment makes cancer less severe without removing the cause, i.e. it does not cure.

Surgery can only remove visible tumours at best and radio- and chemotherapy do more damage to healthy cells, organs, and tissue than to the billions of cancer cells floating around in any patient's body. Therefore, more and more scientists, cancer researchers, medical professionals, as well as patients focus and pin their hopes on immunotherapy.

Cancer vaccines and personalised therapies that eradicate cancer cells and cure the cancer patients for good are intensively researched in many countries and undergo early trials. A lot of work still needs to be done. It is anticipated to take quite a few years before a vaccine or treatment methods like cold atmospheric plasma, collagen disruption to prevent metastasis, or CRISPR will be ready for empirical clinical trials.

For some time, it has been known that the actual cure for cancer exists within each living creature - it is the innate immune system. The question is how this marvellous natural capacity can be strengthened without over-activating it and causing a deadly autoimmune response.

Many attempts have been made and an equivalent number of white blood cell manipulations were pursued in this

200

endeavour. But as is the case with other examples of mankind tampering with nature, most of them had disastrous consequences and resulted in deadly side effects.

It is obvious that more research and a comprehensive understanding of the immune system is needed before an effective cure for cancer in the form of a general immunotherapy will be found.

Consequently, adjunct, adjuvant and orphan medications can serve as a bridging function between conventional and immunotherapies. D,L-methadone has been proven to help making a much-reduced intake of cytotoxic drugs more effective in the apoptosis of all types of cancer cells and tumours. Ketorolac as well as Aspirin have shown in various trials to prevent the recurrence of breast cancer after a surgical intervention. They should receive the financial support needed for intensive research and empirical clinical trials.

Since adjunct and orphan medications only require amounts of as little as 10% of the manufacturers' recommended chemotherapy dosage, Big Pharma will be strictly opposed to any such trials and very likely will not provide any financial assistance to prove their efficacy.

Also, the novel approach of metronomic chemotherapy to administer minute amounts of cytotoxic drugs over a vastly extended period of time should be subjected to an empirical clinical trial to establish beyond a doubt that it can help to cure certain types of cancer with the appropriate chemotherapy.

For good measure, the medicines used by the natives of North America and Siberia to prevent and cure cancer such as Chaga and Smooth Sumac should be intensely investigated to either prove that they provide what is claimed or debunk their anti-cancer properties as a myth.

Finally, other natural substances, such as cannabis, hemp oil, lemon juice, dandelion roots et al, that allegedly have wondrous healing properties, should be compelled to undergo empirical clinical trials as well that should be financed by the producers and vendors of such products. Any of these substances that provide nothing more than a 'feel good effect' should be forced by law to state so clearly and withdraw any claim of anti-cancer properties or the actual healing of any type of cancer.

So, where does that leave the effective immunotherapy that strengthens and enables the immune system to the point of eradicating cancer cells and tumours without doing harm to healthy cells, organs, and tissue? A few promising results have been achieved although the majority of them were effective only for the cancer types leukaemia and melanoma.

Dr. Rosenberg is the standout scientist having achieved a paradigm shift in cancer therapy by strengthening the immune system to the point of it being able to destroy cancer cells and all tumours of a patient with Stage IV cancer without doing harm to healthy cells, organs, and tissue.

Cautiously he warned about his method being highly experimental and very different to any other kind of treatment. Although his method is potentially applicable to any type of cancer, the screening of a patient's white blood cells, extracting those capable of attacking the cancer, growing them in huge quantities in the laboratory, and injecting them into the patient would require the development of a unique drug for every cancer patient.

Prospectively his method will have to be replicated several thousand times before a critical mass of cured cancer patient records can be reviewed and analysed with any hope of finding a common denominator that would allow conclusions for the development of a simplified treatment of all types of cancer and go beyond a unique drug for every cancer patient. Such an analysis would have to include the records of patients whose treatment did not result in the desired outcome of being cured of cancer to establish the 'best case vs. worst case' scenario, which in medical science is not only desirable but also required.

The recent computer technology developments will be of assistance in the analysis of the humongous volume of such medical record data. Considering the time required to accumulate a critical mass of patient records as well as the time to advance quantum computing to a truly useful level, it just may coincide of one being ready for the other.

I hope that in the meantime Dr. Rosenberg will be able to continue his outstanding research work and trials for many years to come.

The scientists who without a doubt will follow in his footsteps and eventually present their effective cancer immunotherapies should be humble enough to acknowledge that they are standing on the shoulders of a giant.

A Few Words of Encouragement

All people diagnosed with cancer who feel that they do not receive the appropriate treatment for their cancer should be given a few words of encouragement:

1. Don't panic or despair - panic and despair cause stress that will make your illness worse

2. Don't give up hope - cancer research is going on all over the world and positive results are not only or necessarily achieved in your country

3. Inform yourself about research results and new treatments - remarkable and scientifically proven results are achieved almost continuously

4. Be persistent when you talk to your doctor and demand explanations that can be understood by a layman

5. Insist on having your questions answered - particularly about the efficacy and cost of the medication your doctor recommends for treatment

6. Learn to differentiate between proven curative medicine and quackery - a qualified doctor willing to prescribe an affordable therapy may be able to help you. Potions, lotions, pills of dubious origin, and all sorts of miraculous treatment options requiring the purchase of exotic and very expensive stuff offered by quacks will not help

7. Be confident and trust your own judgement - not every doctor is a good doctor. If your doctor pooh-poohs scientifically proven curative medications or will not provide medical evidence that supports a diagnosis and you lose trust, say so clearly, and demand a referral

8. Don't be afraid of demanding a second opinion with an institute or doctor that has the latest and best equipment

204

available to permit a detailed review of everything your medical file contains. Your medical reports have to be complete, i.e. not just listing the history of assessments but also a documented diagnosis, a prognosis, and further details such as distressing symptoms that require special care. Based on the outcome of the second opinion decide what steps to take next

9. Remember that only a sick patient is a good patient to the pharmaceutical industry with its costly therapies. If present day anticancer therapies were to heal cancer patients of their disease, the business of each cured patient would be lost and the multi-billion-dollar annual profits would disappear in a puff of smoke

10. Adapt your diet, change to healthy food, and try to give up or at least reduce unhealthy habits. That change of lifestyle also includes more physical activity like long walks or leisurely bicycle rides.

Hopefully these words of encouragement will be of help. Cancer patients should steel themselves mentally and emotionally for a long, tough fight to get the medication they need and can afford.

The following is a list of questions you should ask your doctor about your cancer:

- What kind of cancer do I have?
- Can you show me diagnostic proof and the results of the biopsy that it is the type of cancer you say I have?
- At what stage is my cancer?
- Has the cancer already metastasised?
- What does that mean for my survival?
- What are the treatment or therapy options?
- Which treatment or therapy do you recommend?
- What is the curative effect of the treatment or therapy you recommend?

- What does that treatment or therapy involve?
- What are the side effects of the chemotherapy?
- Do you know metronomic chemotherapy and do you have the equipment and medication to administer it?
- Are any immunotherapies for my type of cancer available in our country? If not, where are they available?
- Will the cost of medication you recommend be covered by the health insurance / universal health care?
- If not, is there any help available to pay for the medication and treatment?
- What medications, treatments and therapies are actually covered by the health insurance / universal health care? Are they any good in your opinion and affordable?
- What clinical trials are going on right now and why would you recommend I join them?
- Where and from whom can I get a second opinion about my diagnosis and treatment options?

That is a long list of questions but you have to insist to have all of them answered in terms of language you can actually understand. Medical shoptalk you should follow up with a demand for clarification in layman's terms.

Add any other questions you may have that will help to put your mind at rest. After all, it is your health and survival that is at stake not the doctor's discomfort of having to answer a lot of questions. Any vague reply or avoidance of giving a clear answer should make you want to ask for a referral.

And finally, inform yourself about your type of cancer as much as possible. Your focus in this endeavour should be on scientific reports whose summaries or conclusions usually provide the answers you want and need in clear and succinct language.

Appendix of Recommended Additional Reading

- Pan-cancer analysis of whole genomes
  The ICGC/TCGA Pan-Cancer Analysis of Whole Genomes, 5th February 2020
  (https://www.nature.com/articles/s41586-020-1969-6)

- Immunotherapy to Treat Cancer
  National Cancer Institute, 28th November 2018
  (https://www.cancer.gov/about-cancer/treatment/types/immunotherapy)

- NCI's Role in Immunotherapy Research
  National Cancer Institute, 19th December 2018
  (https://www.cancer.gov/research/key-initiatives/immunotherapy)

- How Big Pharma Holds Back in the War on Cancer
  Jake Bernstein, ProPublica, 12th July 2017
  (https://www.thedailybeast.com/how-big-pharma-holds-back-in-the-war-on-cancer)

- Availability of evidence of benefits on overall survival and quality of life of cancer drugs approved by European Medicines Agency: retrospective cohort study of drug approvals 2009-13
  Courtney Davis, Huseyin Naci, Evrim Gurpinar, Elita Poplavska, Ashlyn Pinto, Ajay Aggarwal, 4th October 2017
  (http://www.bmj.com/content/359/bmj.j4530)

- Don't Let Big Pharma Make a Killing by Profiteering
  Alex Lawson, Social Security Network, People's Action Blog, 25th March 2020
  (https://www.commondreams.org/views/2020/03/25/dont-let-big-pharma-make-killing-profiteering-covid-19-treatments)

- Report: Most Doctors Receive "Gifts" from Big Pharma
  Ty Bollinger, 8th November 2018
  (https://thetruthaboutcancer.com/gifts-big-pharma/)

- Made in Cuba: A cancer treatment with less toxic side effects
  Tan Shiow Chin, 18th October 2017
  (https://www.star2.com/health/wellness/2017/10/18/ cuban-cancer-treatment-success-story/)

- Facing bleak odds, cancer patients chase one last chance - in Cuba
  Rob Waters, 5th August 2016
  (https://www.statnews.com/2016/08/05/lung-cancer-cuba-biotech/)
- The father of palliative care in Canada, physician Balfour Mount on the legacy of Cicely Saunders, the start of palliative care, and the true meaning of medical aid in dying
  Devon Phillips, 2020
  (https://www.mcgill.ca/palliativecare/portraits-0/balfour-mount)
- MIA In The War On Cancer: Where Are The Low-Cost Treatments?
  Jake Bernstein, ProPublica, 23rd April 2014
  (https://www.propublica.org/article/where-are-the-low-cost-cancer-treatments)
- Methadone as a "Tumor Theralgesic" against Cancer
  Marta Michalska, Arndt Katzenwadel, and Philipp Wolf, University of Freiburg, Germany, October 2017
  (https://www.researchgate.net/publication/320732103_Methadone_as_a_Tumor_Theralgesic_against_Cancer)
- T Cells - Immunotherapy for Treatment of Cancer
  Aida Karachi, 5th November 2018
  (https://www.intechopen.com /books/current-trends-in-cancer-management/immunotherapy-for-treatment-of-cancer)
- B cells - Introductory Chapter: B-Cells
  Mourad Aribi, 26th February 2020
  (https://www.intechopen.com/books/normal-and-malignant-b-cell/introductory-chapter-b-cells)
- NK Cells - NK-cells and Cancer
  May Sabry and Mark W. Lowdell, 13th December 2017
  (https://www.intechopen.com/books/natural-killer-cells/nk-cells-and-cancer)
- CRISPR - What Is CRISPR?
  Minesh Khatri, MD, 14th October 2019
  (https://www.webmd.com/cancer/crispr-facts-overview#1)

- Cold Plasma - Molecular Mechanisms of the Efficacy of Cold Atmospheric Pressure Plasma (CAP) in Cancer Treatment
  Marie Luise Semmler, Sander Bekeschus, Mirijam Schäfer, Thoralf Bernhardt, Tobias Fischer, Katharina Witzke, Christian Seebauer, Henrike Rebl, Eberhard Grambow, Brigitte Vollmar, J. Barbara Nebe, Hans-Robert Metelmann, Thomas von Woedtke, Steffen Emmert and Lars Boeckmann, 2nd December 2019
  (https://www.researchgate.net/publication/338814878_Molecular_Mec hanisms_of_the_Efficacy_of_Cold_Atmospheric_Pressure_Plasma_CA P_in_Cancer_Treatment)

- Perioperative Inflammation as Triggering Mechanism of Metastasis Development
  Michael W. Retsky, Romano Demicheli
  Springer-Nature Book, ISBN-13: 978-3319579429

- Impact of physicians' participation in non-interventional post-marketing studies on their prescription habits: A retrospective 2-armed cohort study in Germany
  Cora Koch, Jörn Schleeff, Franka Techen, Daniel Wollschläger, Gisela Schott, Ralf Kölbel, Klaus Lieb, 26th June 2020
  (https://journals.plos.org/plosmedicine/article?id=10.1371/journal.pme d.1003151)

- Unprovoked Stabilization and Nuclear Accumulation of the Naked Mole-Rat p53 Protein
  Calico Life Sciences LLC, South San Francisco, CA, USA, Marian M. Deuker, Kaitlyn N. Lewis, Maria Ingaramo, Jacob Kimmel, Rochelle Buffenstein & Jeff Settleman
  Sci Rep 10, 6966 (2020). https://doi.org/10.1038/s41598-020-64009-0, 24th April 2020
  (https://www.nature.com/articles/s41598-020-64009-0)

The D,L-methadone aqueous solution recipe

The standard recipe for the racemic D,L-methadone aqueous solution can be presented by anyone to a doctor for a prescription that can be filled by a pharmacist:

- D,L-methadone hydrochloride powder 1.0g
- Ascorbic acid 0.06g
- Citric acid 0.08g
- Aqua purificata ad 100ml
- pipette bottle (important for the constant drop size with 20 drops corresponding to 1ml)

Recommended dosage of D,L-methadone aqueous solution for opioid-naïve patients to be taken sublingually:

Dosing interval = 12 h, optimally ~ 8:00 h & 20:00 h

day 1	- morning and evening	-	5 drops
day 2	- morning and evening	-	10 drops
days 3 to 6	- morning and evening	-	15 drops
from day 7	- morning and evening	-	20 drops

   (equivalent to 1ml for a daily total 2ml or 20mg)

If 2 x 20 drops are well tolerated, dosage can be boosted to 2 x 25 to 2 x 30 drops if needed.

Dr. Hilscher recommends to keep taking D,L-methadone by slowly reducing the dosage for a couple of years after the cancer tumours have been eradicated. It helps to reduce any sign of opioid dependence and prevents the recurrence of cancer.